put
anxiety
behind
you

THE COMPLETE DRUG-FREE PROGRAM

PETER BONGIORNO, ND, LAc

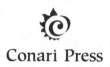

Conari Press

This edition first published in 2015 by Conari Press, an imprint of
Red Wheel/Weiser, LLC
With offices at:
665 Third Street, Suite 400
San Francisco, CA 94107
www.redwheelweiser.com

ISBN: 978-1-57324-630-9

Library of Congress Cataloging-in-Publication Data available upon request

Cover design by Jim Warner
Cover photograph © Miliga / Shutterstock
Author photograph by Inner Source Health
Interior illustrations © Peter Bongiorno
Interior by Jane Hagaman
Typeset in New Baskerville and Gotham Condensed

Printed in Canada
MAR
10 9 8 7 6 5 4 3 2 1

put
anxiety
behind
you

To my courageous patients, who take the less traveled road of natural healing, and to the researchers and clinicians whose tireless and meticulous research work gave this book substance.

contents

acknowledgments

In no way would this work have been completed without the vision and gentle pushes from Caroline Pincus at Red Wheel. Much thanks to Rachel Leach for editing my stream of consciousness into something more readable. Profound gratitude to Patricia Karpas, who started me on this writing journey a few books ago. To my parents, Patricia and Peter, who embody unconditional love, and to the Bongiornos, LoGiudices, Coppolas, and Aunt Rose Zaccaria for providing constant support. My never-ending love goes out to my wife and fellow naturopathic doctor, Pina, the fixed foot who makes my circle just. And to my daughter, Sophia—you inspire me to be my best every day.

disclaimer

This book is not intended as a substitute for professional medical advice. If you are experiencing difficult symptoms of anxiety, please contact a healthcare practitioner, bringing this book with you, if you'd like.

you can do this

We all have a greatest challenge we are working on. This book is special to me, for it allows me to collide, head on, with my strongest challenge and greatest ally—anxiety. And head on is how you and I are going to deal with it for your health, too.

You may be surprised that I called anxiety my greatest ally. Well, it is. Anxiety has helped me make changes that were needed in my life, and I believe anxiety can be your greatest ally and friend, too.

I know you have what it takes.

The very fact that you are reading this book tells me you are ready to face anxiety and move your life forward. Mustering the courage to face this issue squarely is the toughest part and will become its greatest reward. You can do it.

You may have read other books on the subject. You may have seen a psychiatrist or psychologist or two. You may be trying to avoid medications, or you may be on some medications right now. You may think you will never beat this thing. I believed I wouldn't. I can tell you firsthand: you can. You do not have to live the rest of your life in anxiety's grip.

How Is This Book Different?

I am a naturopathic physician. Naturopathic physicians are taught to view health problems from all angles, to look for underlying causes, and to create plans that address these. If there were just one factor causing your anxiety, you would have figured it out already. The truth is there are many factors that uniquely affect your brain and body. These factors then interact with your genetics in such a way to create this syndrome we call anxiety. But genetics are only about 30 percent of the controlling share. The rest of it—the majority of the reasons for your anxiety? You have control over these.

This book gathers about twenty years of my research and eleven years of my clinical practice, and looks at all the factors that contribute to anxiety: lifestyle, diet, sleep, brain chemistry, genetics, and much more. In this book, you and I are going to go over all the things you have control over. I'll outline a clear plan, and give you clear steps help you face anxiety from every angle, in synergy, to truly get to the calm and healing you need and deserve. I will share stories from many other people in your situation, patients of mine who have successfully used these approaches. You will see that you are not alone, and you're not saddled with anxiety—or the medications to treat it—forever. These tools work.

Overall, physical health and good mood are not caused or maintained by any one factor. As I explain to my patients at a first visit, achieving good health is like sitting on a stool. The stool has a number of legs and cross supports that keep it upright and keep you from falling on your butt when you sit down. When one of the legs or supports is weak, your health suffers. The legs you need for getting rid of anxiety for good include:

- Good sleep
- Thought work
- Nutrient and hormonal balance
- Exercise
- Healthy foods
- Healthy digestion
- Blood sugar balance
- Mind-body work
- Supplements

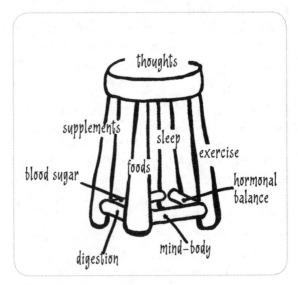

Figure 1.1: The anxiety-free stool

put anxiety behind you

As you can see, the anxiety-free stool has four legs (supplements, foods, exercise, and sleep) and four cross supports (mind-body work, blood sugar balance, healthy digestion, and nutrient and hormone balance)—all supporting a seat of healthy thoughts.

That may sound complicated, but it's really not. It's all about developing awareness of what helps—plus some new habits—and sticking with them. I promise you, if you work on these all together, you will find and maintain your emotional balance.

And by the way, this isn't about being perfect all the time. I do not always eat healthy food. (Trust me, I'm a Sicilian boy at heart who enjoys a good pasta dish or pizza every now and then.) I also occasionally miss days of exercise, and sometimes I miss my supplements. But one thing I have learned is that as long as I keep all of these in mind, and do my best overall, my body and brain reward me. If I go a bit off track with my diet or stay up too late, there is still enough support to keep me up temporarily. And I can get back on track anytime. This process has rewarded me greatly in my journey with anxiety. It will reward you, too.

You can do it! Let's get going . . .

1

what to do right now

Today is a new day.

—Chicken Little

You're probably not feeling so good right now. You may have been diagnosed with generalized anxiety disorder. You may have depression with anxiety, or you may have panic attacks, like I had. You may or may not be taking medications. You just want to put anxiety behind you—preferably forever. I get it. In this short chapter, I will share with you some quick suggestions to help bring things down a notch right away. The rest of the book will give you a more complete view of the factors that contribute to anxiety and offer a way out— but for starters, let's look at some things that can get you feeling better *right now*.

Follow these quick steps, and then start moving through the rest of book at whatever pace you need.

Step 1: Talk to a Doctor
For most people, anxiety is "just anxiety." Nevertheless, it is good to get a general checkup and physical to rule out other health issues that might be contributing to (or even causing) how you feel. Have

your doctor check your blood pressure and ensure that your body is handling the anxiety. If you can see a naturopathic doctor, definitely do so. See appendix II to find a creditable naturopathic doctor or other holistic practitioner.

Ask your medical professional to run some blood work on you. There are specific blood tests that look for odd things that can cause anxiety, like tissues that might abnormally secrete stress hormones. We'll discuss this in more detail in appendix I, which includes a list that you can take to your doctor and an explanation of the blood tests that will uncover other factors that are contributing to your stress. First step: make an appointment for a physical exam. I know this visit alone can cause anxiety for some of you. Nevertheless, when you leave your doctor's office, you will be glad you went.

Step 2: Antianxiety Drugs: Yes or No?

When you go to your doctor and describe how stressed you feel, the subject of antianxiety medications will likely come up. You may already take them.

If you're taking antianxiety medication, even if you don't feel that it is helping, do not abruptly stop taking it. Let your doctor know you'll be trying natural medicines—bring this book along and share it if you like. **Remember, *it is not safe to discontinue medication* without speaking to your doctor first.** Even people who have never been anxious who regularly take these medications for a few months will likely have a hard time stopping cold turkey.

If you believe your medication is helping you, then consider it a blessing. You can start adding in some of the other treatments you'll learn about in this book, and eventually you might try weaning off your medication. ***Under supervision, of course.***

If you're having side effects from your medication and you think the medication is making you feel worse, tell your doctor. He or she may want to adjust the dosage or switch the medication you're taking. Typical side effects of antianxiety medication include memory loss, fogginess, and sleepiness. Some patients will even have physical symptoms like stomach upset, nausea, or problems with coordination. If you are experiencing any of these symptoms, talk to your doctor about discontinuing your medication or switching to another.

If you are not on medication, this simple quiz can help you decide if medication is a good idea for you.

- Does your mood stop you from taking care of yourself to the point where you do not bathe or eat regularly?

- Does your mood stop you from going to work and doing the basic things you need to do for yourself?

- If you have children or dependents, does your mood stop you from taking proper care of them?

- Have you had thoughts of suicide or had the idea that the world would be better off if you were not around?

If you answered "yes" to *any* of the above questions, you should talk with a psychiatrist, physician, or naturopath. I am not a fan of medications and only recommend them as a last resort or in the short term in cases of clear safety concerns. My recommendation would be to look for a licensed naturopathic physician or licensed holistic psychiatrist who can provide medication if needed (see appendix II of this book for resources) while also working with the natural solutions in this book.

If you answered "yes" to the last question and are thinking about hurting yourself, please take action right away. There is a wonderful group of caring people at the National Suicide Prevention Center Lifeline at 1-800-273-TALK (8255)—they want to help. Please call them now.

Step 3: Find Someone to Talk To
Your thoughts are a driving force of your anxiety, and we explore them at length later in this book. But for now, my recommendation is to find a psychologist or therapist with whom you can talk freely. While there is no one best approach, cognitive behavioral therapy (CBT) is considered one of the most effective methods, and it is a good place to start. Consult the Anxiety and Depression Association of America website for a listing of therapists in your area (see appendix II). Also, some wonderful therapists offer Internet-based visits via videoconferencing services like Skype. While I strongly recommend the warmth of an in-person interaction, if your anxiety makes it difficult for you to leave your home or interact directly, a virtual visit might be the place to start.

Step 4: Check In on Sleep

When your sleep is not right, your body naturally gets very anxious.

Sleep has a profound impact on mood. Most people need seven to eight hours per night; some need more. No one really functions well on less. If you are not sleeping enough, do your best to get to bed earlier, preferably before midnight. An ideal sleep schedule is going to sleep at 10:00 p.m. and waking at 6:00 a.m.

While I know many of you reading this are saying "well, that's not for me . . . I'm a night owl," I assure you: you are not an owl. We will work on this in chapter 3. For now, do the best you can to back up your sleep time. If you have a hard time falling asleep, be sure to keep your room as dark as possible at night; avoid the TV, computer, or cell phone for at least a half hour before bed.

Much more about sleep is in chapter 3.

Step 5: Move Your Body

Exercise is nature's way of burning stress hormones. When a dog chases a squirrel, the terrified squirrel's body creates stress hormones and burns them up in the process of running for its life.

Most of us live very inactive lives, yet we are stressed. Our bodies create stress hormones that coarse through us, but we never give ourselves the opportunity to burn them up. It's so important to get up and move:

+ Beginner: thirty minutes of gentle aerobic activity four days a week. This can be broken up into ten-minute increments if you wish—it will still help just as much.

+ Intermediate and advanced: one hour of cardio, with the last thirty minutes being interval training (see chapter 4) four days a week, plus two days of resistance work

Step 6: Balance Blood Sugar

Often when we are stressed out and don't know why, it's because our blood sugar is bouncing all over the place. Time and time again I have seen amazing results come from balancing blood sugar. The short of it is this: when our blood sugar is unstable, the primitive brain sends out a stress response. There is a quick way to fix this.

+ Eat a good breakfast that contains protein, healthy fats, and some healthy carbohydrates every morning. Really. Do it.

- Eat five or six small meals or snacks each day, rather than three big meals. Prepare foods in the morning and carry what you need for the day.

- Add a total of one teaspoon of cinnamon to your food each day. You can add it to cereal, oatmeal—any food, really. Even ketchup tastes good with some cinnamon. More on this in chapter 5.

Step 7: Choose a Mind-Body Modality

When anxiety seems to be controlling you, sometimes you need outside intervention. These are some of my favorite ways to bring the noise down a few decibels:

- Acupuncture, twice a week
- Yoga, every other day
- Massage, once or twice a week
- Reiki, once or twice a week

Step 8: Take These Three Supplements

All of my patients take a triumvirate of supplements that support the body, brain, and digestive tract, while improving production of calming brain neurotransmitters.

1. A high-potency multiple vitamin
2. Fish oil—look for 1,000 mg of eicosapentatoic acid (EPA) a day
3. A probiotic—find a lactobacillus and bifidus combination, yielding about four billion per day

In chapter 7, we will talk more about these basic nutrients for your body and mood. The supplements I use in my clinic can be found on the website *www.3UNeed.com.*

Step 9: Add These Antianxiety Supplements

There are many supplements for anxiety out there. In my practice, I have often found the following supplements to be as effective as medications, but with fewer side effects.

- For generalized anxiety, start with a lavender gelcap supplement.
- For panic attacks, use the lavender supplement and add one teaspoon of glycine and one-half teaspoon of passionflower extract three times a day.

- For issues related to obsessive-compulsive disorder, use the supplements listed above, plus 500 mg of n-acetyl cysteine three times a day, away from food (twenty minutes before a meal or at least one hour after a meal).

- For anxiety with depression, try 100 mg of 5-hydroxy-tryptophan (5-HTP) three times a day along with 300 mg of St. John's wort three times a day. If taking other medications, check with your doctor or pharmacist before starting St. John's wort, for this herb can interfere with other drugs.

In chapter 7, we will take a closer look at the supplements discussed in the last two steps, as well as a number of others.

I hope you have found this brief sketch helpful. If you are struggling to put one foot in front of the other or even to get out of bed, these suggestions can be a real lifeline. Next, we'll loop back to the beginning and explore what anxiety is and how and why it happens.

2

your thoughts

The cave you fear to enter holds the treasure you seek.
—Joseph Campbell

Case: Linda with Breast Cancer

Linda was a fifty-eight-year-old lawyer who originally came to see me for support during breast cancer treatment. She had already had a lumpectomy and was looking for care to help support her body during chemotherapy and radiation treatments. Together, we outlined a strong diet to help her body stay healthy, discussed strategies for better sleep hygiene, and selected nutrient supplements for overall health. Linda came to visit me for regular acupuncture on a weekly basis to complement her naturopathic care. During her cancer treatments, she did beautifully—and felt she was healthier than others in her treatment group. She stayed energetic, upbeat, and in a way felt better than ever.

But once Linda's chemotherapy treatment was finished, she felt "unprotected." Life began to feel dark and anxious. This is a common reaction in patients who have just finished cancer treatment. Linda's sleep suffered. She told me about her anxieties regarding her relationship with her husband, which had been strained for many years—he had cheated on her once or twice. Linda forgave her husband because they had three children whose lives she did not want to disrupt. She also did not think she could make it financially on her own. She felt trapped and powerless.

We talked about her self-esteem and how relationship issues can settle, energetically, in breast tissue—the area of nurture. I recommended that Linda read books on self-esteem and start considering what was important about life. While her conventional doctors recommended antianxiety drugs, I recommended that she face her issues head on. We also started some herbal remedies, such as St. John's wort and rhodiola, as well as tryptophan for sleep.

While this was a difficult time for Linda, it also became a time of empowerment. Eventually, she was able to confront her husband, who had his own issues of anxiety. For the first time, she was living her "real life." Linda realizes that the breast cancer was an unfortunate wake-up call that ended up helping her more than anything had before.

This book is about healing from anxiety and taking back full control of your life. To do this, we need to address the physical part of you—your sleep, your digestion, your foods and nutrients. Most of this book is designed to do that.

While most of this book deals with your physical body to help calm your brain, this chapter looks at the thoughts that drive anxiety and gives you the tools to start working on them. Chapter 8 will help you design a plan to challenge the anxiety when you are ready.

For me, anxiety was the catalyst that led to the lowest points of my life. As you probably know, anxiety and panic attacks are truly frightening. At times, my feelings of dread, nausea, and overall ugliness were more than I could bear. Even more, the toll anxiety took on my life was profound: I was unable to do certain things because of anxiety, and I felt ashamed and embarrassed. It woefully lowered my self-esteem.

Does this all sound familiar to you?

If so, that is good.

Huh? Did I say that was a "good" thing?

Yes, I did. Because if it's in you to feel that scared, that fearful, that embarrassed—then you can feel that *great*, too. The same mechanisms that cause you to fully feel the anxiety, also allow you to feel happy and excited about life. It is completely in you to feel your best—your body can do it.

Why do I know you can do it? Because your mind is imaginatively creating anxiety. If it can do that, then it can create a life without it, too. One of the best pieces of information I was given when I started my anxiety journey was that *I* was the creator of my anxiety—and I could uncreate it, too. Up until that point, I thought external factors caused my anxiety or that there was something wrong with my brain. Actually, my brain worked well—a little too well.

You know how some people love riding roller coasters, while others hate them? Why is that? Well, when a roller slowly brings you up to the top of the drop and you expect to plunge down at breakneck speed, what happens in your body?

Your Stress System: the HPA Axis and Allostatic Load

Before we move any farther, I want to briefly explain the stress system. This way, as you read this and other books, you will have a good framework to make sense of it all.

Any time you are excited or threatened, a part of your brain called the cerebral cortex responds. This is the outside surface of the brain—the part that makes humans different from all the other animals. The cerebral cortex decides right there: "Hey, this is gonna be fun" or "Hey, this is dangerous; I think I might die here."

Whichever it is, that input gets sent into the middle of the brain—the hypothalamus. This brain center is where your immune system, nervous system, and hormonal system meet up to coordinate responses. From the hypothalamus, the signal goes to the bottom part of the brain, the pituitary, which sends a signal to tiny glands on the top of the kidneys called the adrenal glands. These adrenal glands are responsible for emitting stress hormones like epinephrine and norepinephrine (also known as "adrenaline" in England and other parts of the world). Epinephrine is the hormone that causes you to react and feel afraid (by raising your heartrate and increasing sweating, muscle tightening, tingling, and so on—all the feelings you know so well). Norepinephrine helps you focus on the threat—so you keep feeling anxious. Cortisol is another stress hormone that moves blood sugar and makes you hungry. Cortisol also beats up on your brain tissue, giving you that surreal and floaty feeling medical professionals call "depersonali-

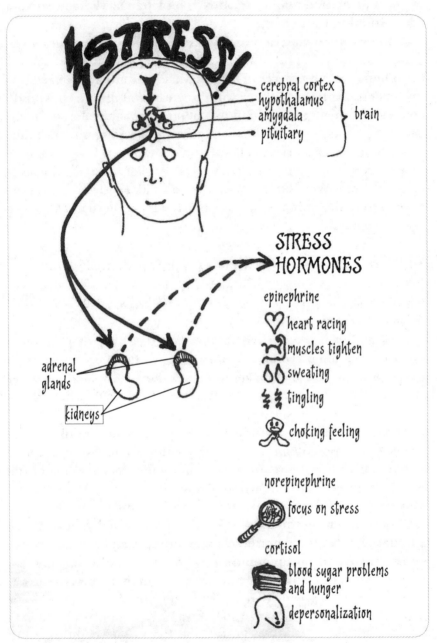

Figure 2.1: The hypothalamic pituitary adrenal response system

put anxiety behind you

zation." The hypothalamus may share signals with the amygdala, a fear center in the brain that can help coordinate and enhance the sensation of fear and panic. This system is called the Hypothalamic Pituitary Adrenal response system (HPA). Below is a diagram to help you follow this.

In the short term, the release of stress hormones readies your body for action—to fight or to run. This reaction can save your life. In the long term, however, this reaction can cause imbalances in your system. High levels of epinephrine, norepinephrine, and cortisol make it difficult for the body to keep up.

In the 1920s, Hungarian endocrinologist Hans Selye conducted research on a condition he called general adaptation syndrome (GAS). Selye realized that the stress response that can save your life can become a problem if it goes on too long. Let's say a bear is coming at you. At first, you have a stress response called the alarm reaction—your body creates stress hormones, and you run from that bear. But let's say the bear doesn't let up—it chases you for days and days. You start to adapt to it—you get used to that bear chasing you to the point where it feels almost normal. It's sort of like a little Volkswagen that is running RPMs in the red—it may be able to do so in the short term to push past a tractor-trailer on the highway, but you can't run a car like that all the time.

Your body has a similar reaction to stress. Like the little Volkswagen, you end up "running out of gas" and break down, feeling anxious and depleted. In the 1990s, researcher Bruce McEwen teased out this issue further by documenting the unhealthy changes to the body that occur with long-term stress: McEwen noted changes in blood pressure, cholesterol, blood sugar, inflammation, and many other body processes. You get used to running in the red for a while, but over time, the body breaks down. Most of my patients with anxiety have been in the red for a while or are starting to break down. The adrenal saliva test described in appendix I can help your doctor understand where you are on the stress continuum.

General Adaptation Syndrome:
Healthy Balance → Alarm Reaction → Adaptation → Burnout

Back to the Thoughts

Now that we have a little stress physiology under our belts, let's get back to the thoughts that push this physiology with a question: How come some people love wild roller coaster rides, while others are scared of them? It all starts with your thoughts! You have the mechanism to be anxious or to enjoy life—it really is up to you in the end. The key is changing the thought and retaking control of what you're thinking. While the rest of this book will focus on what you can do for your body to reduce anxiety, this chapter focuses directly on changing those thoughts.

While I know it may not sound possible right now, this is something you can do. Remember, if you have the mechanism to be afraid, you also have the mechanism to enjoy life and move through anxiety!

Your Hero's Journey

> We're in a free-fall into future. We don't know where we're going. Things are changing so fast, and always when you're going through a long tunnel, anxiety comes along. And all you have to do to transform your hell into a paradise is to turn your fall into a voluntary act. It's a very interesting shift of perspective and that's all it is . . . joyful participation in the sorrows and everything changes.
>
> —Joseph Campbell

I have already quoted Joseph Campbell twice in this chapter. I first came across Campbell's work as a high school student in the mid-1980s, when I saw the *Power of Myth* series on PBS. Filmed over a few days at George Lucas's Skywalker Ranch, the program features Bill Moyers in conversation with Joseph Campbell. In this interview, Campbell discusses a concept called the "hero's journey" and relates it to both ancient civilizations and our modern world.

Like the typical teenager, I was preoccupied with superficial fancies, but Campbell's words mesmerized me. They started me on a path to think more deeply and completely about my life and what made me happy.

In case you don't know who this fellow is, let me fill you in: Joseph Campbell was a mythologist who lived from 1904 to 1987. As a mythologist, he spent time trying to understand the different religions, philosophies, and stories ("myths") as told in various cultures, art, and literature from around the world.

What Campbell learned from his collected research was that many cultures and civilizations that had no communication with one another (no Internet, no Facebook, no Snapchat or Twitter—maybe carrier pigeons, but that's about it) had many similar ideas about the universe, God, and religion. Campbell found that even though these civilizations did not communicate, many of them independently honored the theme of "the hero."

The typical hero (or heroine) story was about someone who may have lived a normal life for a time, went through a great challenge, and somehow came out on the other side transformed. Because these heroes are not looking to be heroic and usually feel out of place where they are, they experience anxiety of their own. At the end of the story, the hero always ends up wiser and is restored to an even higher sense of self and purpose in the world.

Famous examples of the hero's journey include major figures from world religions, such as Buddha, Moses, Mohammed, and Jesus. Classic literature also carries the hero theme—there is the character of Odysseus from the *Odyssey* or Stephen in James Joyce's *Portrait of the Artist as a Young Man*. Popular culture repeats the same beautiful theme with characters like Dorothy from the *Wizard of Oz*, Harry Potter, Disney's Mulan, Spiderman, and Luke Skywalker from *Star Wars*.

What I am trying to get at is that **you are the hero or heroine, too!** Don't look around the room—I am talking to you . . . yes, you.

We need to talk about the challenges you are facing, how to think about them as a part of the hero's journey, and how to get you to the other side. From now on, you are not a vulnerable person facing insurmountable problems. Rather, you are someone with challenges that can be

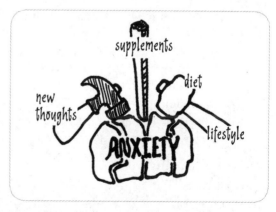

Figure 2.2: Breaking up anxiety

worked through. As you read through this book, you will work on both your physical body, which can drive anxious thoughts, as well as the thoughts themselves. Working from both sides is the best way to break up and get rid of anxiety for good.

Today, maybe for the first time, you are going to summon the hero you have in you—the hero we have in all of us—and learn to move through the murky darkness into a new light of understanding, a light of calm, love, and greatly reduced anxiety.

How to Change Your Thoughts in Three Steps

To help with this metamorphosis, we will focus on three steps.

1. Bring in new information
2. Write it, rate it, and change the thought
3. Think like a Buddhist

Step 1: Bring In New Information

There's an old saying someone told me when I started this journey for myself: "Keep doing the same thing to keep getting the same results." Similarly, if you keep thinking the same thoughts, you will continue to invoke the fear reaction you have been dealing with all this time.

At one point in my life, I thought I couldn't ride on an airplane anymore. In fact, I was sure of it. These feelings were so strong—the panic was too overwhelming. But in the long run, it turns out that the thought was wrong—and I was wrong. These days I fly all the time, giving lectures and traveling for fun. I worked on changing my thoughts about airplane rides, and you can change your thoughts, too.

The first step to changing your anxiety is to start bringing in other ideas. This isn't really any different than working with other disease states. Often, I work with patients who are very sick due to toxic accumulation in their bodies—toxins like pesticides, plastics, unhealthy fats, excess calories, heavy metals, chemicals from the environment, and foods to which they are very sensitive. These toxins can cause many types of sickness: autoimmune diseases, cancers, heart disease, diabetes, and skin problems, to name a few. Essentially, these toxins provide bad information to the body—they tell the cells to stay unhealthy.

put anxiety behind you

The best way to counteract toxic accumulations is to nourish the body with new foods and good information. Foods such as blueberries, mercury-free fish, organic carrots, organic green vegetables, and organic olive oils have the opposite effect—they send positive messages to our cells. Similarly, to change anxiety, you will need to change the messages that go to your brain's prefrontal cortex. The messages we tell ourselves make all the difference.

I had a teenage patient who came to see me with her mom. She was sixteen years old and had suffered from anxiety for the past year. We talked about her diet, sleep, stressors, and the right nutrients for her brain. I explained to my patient that changing the messages in the brain is like "a cassette tape, playing a negative message over and over." I suggested that she "erase that tape—and record a new one." She looked perplexed—she did not know what a cassette tape was. So we switched it to an MP3 on her phone, and she understood—whew!

Whether it's on a cassette tape or an MP3, we have to start bringing in new messages—messages that look at the roller coaster and say "hey—that looks fun" versus "I am going to die." Now, I am not saying that you have to go on a roller coaster. Whatever your personal roller coaster is, you have to "transform that hell into a paradise." It is within you to do this.

It was helpful for me to read different books that sent me new messages. I learned that no one book is going to do it. This is certainly one of those books, but as you take your hero's or heroine's journey, I want you to look for more. Go to the bookstore (yes . . . I know the bookstore is a vanishing breed, but it is much more charming than Amazon), take a look at some books and videos, see which ones resonate with you, and start with those.

Here are a few of my favorites. Please note some do not necessarily focus on the theme of anxiety, but they bring out themes that are super important.

Taking the Leap. Pema Chödrön was the first Western female to become a Buddhist monk. This book is short, but thick with insight and peaceful beauty. Read this one slowly, chapter by chapter. Read it twice.

How We Choose to Be Happy: The 9 Choices of Extremely Happy People—Their Secrets, Their Stories. Foster and Hicks's book discusses how happy people think and the choices they make.

Accepted (film). This is a favorite movie of mine that uses comedy to reveal the importance of being who you are and realizing that the greatest opportunities will come when you follow your passions.

The Power of Myth (film). These recordings of Bill Moyers's interviews with Joseph Campbell allow you to hear, in Campbell's own words, how to look at literature and art in the context of your own life's journey.

How to Make Yourself Happy and Remarkably Less Disturbable. Albert Ellis's classic book is a favorite among psychologists. It explains how to use your natural ability to think positively.

The Hero with a Thousand Faces. Joseph Campbell's 1949 book describes the hero's journey and gives examples throughout literature and art.

Feel the Fear and Do It Anyway. Susan Jeffers's practical book is about how to think about anxiety and move through it.

Ferris Bueller's Day Off (film). A classic comic movie not just for those who like to ditch school. Ferris Bueller is really about letting go of the mundane in order to appreciate life to its fullest.

From Panic to Power. Lucinda Bassett's book is an excellent guide to accepting anxiety, instead of running from it, as a means to move through it successfully. A wonderful primer on changing thoughts.

Overcome Your Fear of Driving. Rich Presta's self-help program is a valuable resource for anyone with a specific fear of driving. Presta uses a commonsense approach combined with anxiety-busting ideas from many other approaches to create a program that can really help you get back on the road. While focused on driving, it can apply to any anxiety or situational fear.

Rio (film). Animated film about a bird who faces a fear of flying. The main character, Blu, finds something more important in life than his fear.

Talladega Nights: The Ballad of Ricky Bobby (film). Starring Will Ferrell, this offbeat movie explores a racecar driver's work to face his fear of driving after an accident. I can't stop laughing about this one—and it's hard to be anxious when you're laughing that hard.

Why People Don't Heal, and How They Can. Carolyn Myss's book and audiotape from 1998 dives into emotional baggage and how it holds us back. Myss has an excellent four-disc CD set entitled *Self Esteem: Your Fundamental Power* that gets to the heart of anxiety and lack of self-esteem.

I also have thoroughly enjoyed Oprah Winfrey's "Life Class," which can be accessed on her website. By the way, Oprah Winfrey is a very successful person who has overcome her own severe anxiety as part of her journey, and now her mission is to support others in their journeys.

Step 2: Write It, Rate It, and Change the Thought

Write It

The alcoholic's main issue is clear—too much drinking. Do you know the first step the alcoholic takes toward recovery? Recognizing and admitting that he or she is drinking too much. Some alcoholics don't even realize they are going for that drink. The habit has become so ingrained, they aren't even conscious of what they are doing. So the first step is that simple—just notice when you take a drink.

Like alcoholics, those of us who are anxious move to anxious thoughts without even realizing we are doing it! Even though we always have a choice, we default to anxiety. I remember I used to wake up in the morning, and already the negative messages were buzzing:

"This is going to be a bad day."

"I won't be able to get everything done that I need to."

"I will probably fail at what I want to do."

"I am not smart or talented enough to achieve my goals."

"I am too anxious to succeed."

There's no way in the world someone can succeed if they are thinking that way. Let me ask you a question. If you were my patient, and every time you came to see me I told you that you were a bad person, or a loser, or a jerk, would you come back to me for help? If I hit you in the head with an emotional baseball bat and beat you up during every visit, would you return for more visits and more abuse?

No, of course not. But when you have anxious thoughts, you are doing that to yourself. You are keeping the anxiety going. When we are angry or scared, we bottle it up inside us until it comes out as anger and negative thinking. This negative thinking has to stop.

How can you stop it? The first step is recognizing it when it happens. Pick up a notebook or find a spot on your cell phone where you can make a note every time you catch yourself having a negative thought. Do it throughout the day for the next two days. When I first did this exercise, my hand hurt because I was writing all day!

I have noticed that when I ask my patients to do this, some people will make a note in their head but not physically write it down. While noting in your head is a first step, it is not enough to accomplish your goals. So don't just think about it—write it down. This is key.

Why write it? Many famous writers have weighed in on the power of recording your thoughts. One smart person after another has said the same thing about writing:

> *How do I know what I think until I see what I say?*
> —E. M. Forster

> *Writing has got to be an act of discovery . . .*
> *I write to find out what I'm thinking about.*
> —Edward Albee

> *I never know what I think about something*
> *until I read what I've written on it.*
> —William Faulkner

> *I write entirely to find out what I'm thinking.*
> —Joan Didion

> *I write because I don't know what I think until I read what I say.*
> —Flannery O'Connor

> *I don't know what I think until I write it down.*
> —Norman Mailer

I think you get the point—and research backs this up. Basically, if you write down the thoughts and then read them, you will be able to process them through more parts of your brain and create a better perspective. When you have a better perspective, things feel less scary, and you are more amenable to positive change.

Rate It

Once you have written your thought, I want you to give it a score, from one to ten, of how strong it is for you. A one is a pretty weak thought that doesn't cause much anxiety. A ten is very strong—your anxiety is through the roof.

Change the Thought

Once you have rated your anxious or negative message, the next step is to ask yourself whether it is really true. If it is true, you can make a realistic plan to fix the problem. If it is not true (most are not), write down a more positive thought. Here are some examples:

"This is going to be a bad day." 7/10

Is this true? No.

The new thought: No one has a crystal ball, and I am sure there will be good aspects to this day.

"I won't be able to get everything done that I need to." 5/10

Is this true? Yes.

The new thought: I might be doing way too many things—more than any one person can do. I will prioritize my tasks and be okay with whatever I *can* do. The things that don't get done? Well, I will get to them tomorrow.

"I will probably fail at what I want to do." 4/10

Is this true? No.

The new thought: I do many things well. I can only try my best today. Anything that doesn't go well I can learn from and use it to my advantage to do even better tomorrow.

"I am not smart or talented enough to succeed." 8/10

Is this true? No.

The new thought: Actually, I am a smart person with many strengths.

"I am too anxious to be successful." 9/10

Is this true? No.

The new thought: Most successful people are actually anxious people. I can control my anxiety and use it to my advantage.

And, by the way—it is completely true that anxious people tend to be successful, smart, and creative. Abraham Lincoln had serious anxiety. The famous singers Adele and Barbra Streisand have terrible stage fright and phobias. The soccer star David Beckham is known to have obsessive-compulsive disorder. Whoopi Goldberg had a tremendous fear of flying. As I mentioned, Oprah Winfrey fashioned her personal anxieties to her advantage and has become one of the most successful business and entertainment personalities of all time.

When anxiety is controlled, it can help you stay alert and interested. We are not going to rid you of 100 percent of your anxiety—for some anxiety is good to keep you sharp and focused. We are just redirecting the anxiety when it becomes debilitating. I have realized that I am an anxious person—and that is okay as long as I have compassion for myself and use the anxiety to better myself rather than stopping myself. When anxiety stops me, I work on changing the thought.

What about Scary Thoughts?
Much of the time, people with anxiety have scary thoughts. They think they are going to lose control or that they will embarrass themselves by not being able to handle a situation. Even more, they may have fleeting thoughts about hurting themselves or others. There may even be a moment when they think it would be easier if they were not around. If you are having scary thoughts like this, it is always good idea to check in with a psychologist or counselor.

Typically, though, my anxious patients who have scary thoughts do not act on them. In fact, they do just the opposite. If you ask an anxious person to stop in the middle in the road and go berserk, he will not do it—he is too embarrassed! This illustrates how your scary thoughts are just manifestations of your creative mind running amok. They are part of the anxiety cascade that is attempting to take over your life. Like spoiled kids, they want your attention—and the more attention you give them, the more they act up. Don't give them too much attention—just check in with someone, then move on to step 3.

Step 3: Think Like a Buddhist
First, let me say that I am not suggesting that you have to become a Buddhist.

I do want to explain, though, that much of my own anxiety came from two sources: trying to distract myself from things I did not want to think about in my own life, and a simple fear of death. Learning about Buddhist ways of thinking helped me lessen my anxiety and get on with life.

My anxiety and panic attacks first surfaced when I was in my early twenties. At the time, I was a drummer playing in an unsuccessful rock band. I was having fun but living a stressful and pretty unhealthy life. I had a pretty scary spinout on the highway, and I experienced the traumatic breakup of a relationship that I thought would last forever. I started having trouble driving on the highway and even difficulty walking on train platforms. Talk about scary thoughts—I kept thinking I would purposely jump onto the tracks and get run over by an oncoming train. Playing the drums was my favorite thing to do, but even that suffered. I started to get stage fright—I would get dizzy and lose my timing on stage and during recording. If you know anything about the drums, losing your timing is a disaster. Things that were once simple and enjoyable—driving, playing the drums, and riding the train—were all being taken away from me. Fear of flying in an airplane naturally followed.

Anxiety is a lot like the alien from *The Blob*. Remember that movie? It's a science fiction and horror film from 1958 about an alien amoeba that comes to a small Pennsylvania town and feeds on citizens and property. The more it consumes, the larger the creature grows. Once the Blob gets a hold on something, it wants to take more and more. A twenty-seven-year-old Steve McQueen figures out the blob's weakness—the cold. The townspeople use fire extinguishers to beat back and defeat the alien.

My "anxiety blob" took up more and more of my life, and I allowed it to flourish. That is, until I figured out anxiety's weakness: reframing my thoughts and taking care of my health!

Looking back, I know there were a few reasons for my anxiety—but believe it or not, my traumatic breakup, car spinout, and unsuccessful rock band were not the culprits! These were only the excuses I focused on to distract myself. No person or situation was the cause of my anxiety. I needed to take responsibility, but I was not ready to do so.

The real reasons for my anxiety? These were lack of sleep and exercise, poor diet, and, even more, I was worried about my future, and I was scared of death. Once I took responsibility for these things and stopped blaming others, the anxiety was greatly diminished.

What situations or people do you blame for your anxiety? Are these feelings distracting you from taking responsibility for your life and moving forward?

My anxiety blob made me aware that something was out of balance, and it distracted me from more important issues. It is likely that *your* anxiety blob is born from a number of physical and emotional issues that need your attention. This book will help identify those issues.

In Buddhism, there's a saying that "all suffering comes from attachment." When you think about it, it is true. When a loved one passes away, we are sad, because we want that person with us. Of course it is understandable to feel sad and mourn that loss. When I broke up with my girlfriend, I suffered because I was attached to her and to the idea that she would be with me forever. I was also attached to the idea of playing music as a means of making money and being happy. When I started to realize that it might not work out that way, and that I didn't have control of the outcomes I was attached to, I suffered and became anxious. The lack of sleep, lack of exercise, and poor food choices increased the negative feelings even more.

What about that airplane anxiety? What was I attached to there? Well, it was another manifestation of my creative mind working against me and exaggerating my fear of death. I wanted to stay on this earth. I thought about hurtling through space at hundreds of miles an hour, and I didn't want to die in a metal cylinder like that. More than likely, if you have anxiety, I'll bet flying in that airplane doesn't make you feel too good either—but you can move through it. What Buddhism has helped me understand is that life itself will come and go. This isn't necessarily a good or bad thing. It just is what it is.

I know what I am about to say might sound a bit strange or maybe even insulting. But I am going to say it anyway: fear of death, in some ways, is simply arrogant and egotistical. Why? Because we think of ourselves as so important to this earth that it would be a tragedy if we left this world. But in reality, no matter who we are, we will pass on, and the world will go on without us. If this is true, why get anxious about it? Sure, if I was crushed by a falling piano on my way home from the office, I am sure my family would be sad. But the truth is, they would go on . . . and they would be okay. To tell you the truth, I am not sure I am fully without fear of death 100 percent, but at least I don't think about it all the time the way I used to. Hypochondria doesn't control my life the way it did. Now, rather than worrying about death, I just enjoy more of the moment.

In fact, if you really are in the present moment, it is impossible to be anxious. Anxiety is all about being worried about the future or being upset about the past. The present moment is incompatible with anxiety. This is why we discuss meditation in chapter 6.

A good book to get started with Buddhism is *Why I Am a Buddhist* by Stephen Asma. It is a great book for those who want to stay away from the New Age feel that can scare off a lot of people. This book touts its ability to avoid "New Age mush" and "does not require a diet of brown rice, burning incense, and putting both your mind and your culture in deep storage." Another good book is Thubten Chodron's *Buddhism for Beginners,* which explains Buddhist concepts plainly and with gentle balance. Please add these books to your new thoughts book list.

Let's Recap

Step 1. Bring in new information. Check out the list of books and films to get started.

Step 2. Write it, rate it, and change it. Start writing down your thoughts in bullet form and rate them on a scale of 1 to 10 (10 causing the most anxiety). Write down a thought that counters the scary thought. Do this for every negative thought you catch yourself having.

Step 3. Think like a Buddhist. Pick up one of the Buddhism books mentioned. Start to unattach and remain in the present moment.

3

sleep

Sleep that knits up the raveled sleave of care,
The death of each day's life, sore labor's bath,
Balm of hurt minds, great nature's second course,
Chief nourisher in life's feast.
                                        —*Macbeth,* act II, scene II

Case: Candice with Early Perimenopausal Sleep Issues and Anxiety

Candice was forty-two years old and never had an anxious day in her life. She originally came into my office because of chronic knee issues, which we were able to resolve with weight loss, acupuncture, orthotics, and strengthening exercises. When Candice walked into my office four years later, her gait was fine, but she looked haggard: bloodshot eyes, pale, and sluggish. "I haven't slept in two months," she said. For the past six months, she and her husband had been trying to get pregnant with their second child. Unfortunately, no luck. And now there was definitely no chance—if she wasn't getting any sleep, she wasn't up for sex, either. Even more, she was starting to have daily bouts of anxiety, especially in bed: palpitations, sweats, and general "electric buzzing," as she put it.

After taking a thorough history and running some labs, I determined that there were probably a few factors at play. Candice shared how she was under a lot of stress at work, a job she had had for six years. When she finally came home at night (which was often after six o'clock.), she only had an hour or so to spend with her six-year-old daughter before her daughter's bedtime. Then she had a lot of errands that kept her on the computer and running around up until bedtime, when she collapsed with exhaustion, maybe attempted to have intercourse, and then stared at the ceiling in "tired and wired" fashion. I ran some saliva tests that showed high nighttime cortisol and low progesterone, which her blood work also corroborated. Her B vitamins, iron, and vitamin D were also low, suggesting she was generally depleted.

When women move into their forties, it is not uncommon that progesterone, the hormone needed for the second half of the menstrual cycle and to help carry pregnancy, will start to drop. High stress makes it drop even faster. Low progesterone will drop GABA, a neurotransmitter the brain needs to stay calm and sleep.

I started Candice with some good sleep rituals, established a regular bedtime schedule, and placed her on some time-release melatonin, phosphatidylcholine, and nighttime progesterone. The melatonin helps the body naturally know what time it is, the phosphatidylcholine helps to gently lower cortisol, and progesterone restores proper activity of GABA. We also talked about eating more nourishing foods, like vegetable and fish soups, and taking some high-potency multiple vitamins. Within two weeks, her sleep had improved dramatically, and her anxiety was almost gone.

Once Candice's sleep began to improve, we started to talk about the root causes of her insomnia and what her body was trying to tell us. We discussed how her work schedule and all that stress made it hard to create the room needed to bring another baby into the world. Candice rearranged her priorities and started a yoga and meditation plan. These changes were

put anxiety behind you

key to lowering her daytime anxiety, and they reduced that "wired" feeling. At age forty-three, Candice became pregnant, then gave birth to another healthy baby girl.

If you have insomnia, I want to tell you—you can sleep again. There is an exceedingly rare condition called fatal familial insomnia that you have less than a one in a million chance of getting. Unless you have this disease (which I have never seen in my years of working with patients), you can fix your sleeping issues. Candice learned that without good sleep, anxiety comes on quite easily. As the Shakespeare quote at the beginning of the chapter describes, even a seventeenth-century playwright keenly realized the importance of sleep as something that cures your aches and relaxes your anxious mind.

If you are an anxious person and sleep well, congratulate yourself! You are in the minority. In fact, if you sleep well, you can skip this chapter—just make sure that if your schedule allows, you are getting to bed by eleven o'clock and waking up seven-plus hours later. If you are going to bed much later (and do not work the night shift—see more on that later), then I still need you to read this chapter.

I've included a whole chapter on sleep because I have seen over and over again the effects that sleep (or lack thereof) have on anxiety and mood. In this chapter, we will work through your symptoms and come up with a plan to get you to sleep.

A January 2014 study by the Centers for Disease Control found that around sixty million Americans have sleep disorders, making our sleep deprivation a real "public epidemic." Sleep and anxiety almost always go hand in hand. Most people with anxiety have sleep issues. And most of the time, if you don't sleep well, you are going to be more anxious—the worse the sleep, the worse the anxiety the following day. As a physician, I spend a good deal of time trying to figure out how to help my patients sleep.

All animals—humans included—require sleep. Lack of proper sleep can increase the risk of viral colds, weight gain, poor memory, and cognitive problems. A study published in the *Archives of Internal Medicine* showed that less than seven hours of sleep raises the risk of contracting respiratory viral illness by 300 percent over those who get eight or more hours of sleep. More importantly for you, sleep deprivation increases anxiety directly by causing inflammation, as well as hormonal and blood sugar imbalances.

"But I'm a Night Owl!"

Many of my patients will say, "I'm not a morning person . . . I'm a night owl. I am super tired during the day, but then I wake up and feel well in the evening."

Does this describe you? If so, you are not alone. As described earlier, my anxiety first presented itself when I was in my early twenties and playing in a rock band. At the time, I swore I was a night owl. I'd be up at all hours into the early morning, and then sleep off most of the day, waking up at three or four in the afternoon. Then I'd be *exhausted* all day and wonder why—after all, I was getting eight to eleven hours of sleep. I also did not have a clue that there was a strong correlation between my anxiety and my sleeping patterns.

Today I know that excess stress (like trying to make it in a rock band and struggling to pay rent) and excess exposure to nighttime bright light and activity (like being on stage at a nightclub) can disrupt sleep patterns and cause a condition called delayed sleep phase syndrome (DSPS). People with this condition feel the need to go to sleep later and later in the evening. DSPS is not well known, but it is a fairly common cause of insomnia.

The pineal gland of the brain secretes the hormone melatonin as the darkness of night approaches. When darkness hits your eyes, they send signals to the pineal to make melatonin. Melatonin tells your body "hey, it is time to sleep." It prepares your nervous system for sleep by lowering body temperature and inducing drowsiness. Melatonin is also powerful antioxidant known to help your body fight cancer, detoxify, and boost the immune system.

If your brain is not putting melatonin out at the right time in the early evening, sleep architecture gets messed up, and your mood suffers. If the melatonin is inappropriately secreted, you can end up with a circadian rhythm problem. Appendix I describes saliva cortisol testing and how normal circadian rhythms are super important for healthy brain function and mood.

A characteristic symptom of DSPS is the feeling that you can't fall asleep. This is known as sleep onset insomnia. Other common and equally troubling issues are waking up a several times per night, or waking up too early in the morning. DSPS sufferers end up feeling like night owls—they are up most of the night and have a hard time falling asleep and staying asleep. As a result, they are exhausted the next day or "wired and tired"—anxious and wired up, but still exhausted at the same time. Some of my patients tell me that when they finally start falling asleep in the wee hours of the morning, they have to get up for work. Once they are awake, they experience debilitating fatigue and anxiety during the day. By the time the night rolls around, they experience a "second wind" that keeps the bad sleep cycle going. I see this issue with many of my high school age patients. In fact, up to 10 percent of high school students have DSPS and suffer chronic sleep deprivation.

"I Can't Stay Asleep" or "I Wake Up Way Too Early"

Even if you are able to fall asleep, you might struggle to *stay asleep* during the course of the night. Or you may have issues with waking up way too early (somewhere in the range of three or four in the morning) and then feeling wired. If you are lucky, you might get up and feel fine for a few hours, but then slip into great anxiety and tiredness for the rest of the day. Some people wake up with a tremendous panicky anxiety and simultaneous fatigue; others experience early morning nausea and/or vomiting or a disturbingly stuffy nose. No matter your symptoms, it's a rough way to start the new day.

Rapid eye movement (REM) sleep is a component of the last stage of sleep that occurs in both animals and people. Known as "dream sleep," this stage tends to be very light and active. While it's normal for newborn babies to spend about 80 percent of their sleep in REM, adults shouldn't experience more than 25 percent REM sleep. Because the brain's processing activity is similar to the type experienced in waking moments, the more REM sleep you experience, the less refreshing your sleep will be.

Chances are that if you have anxiety, then you probably have much more REM sleep than deep, "slow wave" sleep. People with anxiety tend to enter REM sleep unusually early in the sleep cycle, have an extended first REM phase, and spend less time in the slow wave sleep phase. If you have a hard time staying asleep and you wake up way too early, this is you.

Why All the REM Sleep?

I believe at some level, your brain and body are trying to help you work out the anxiety.

During the day, there are great distractions: family, work, school—even anxiety is a distraction. At nighttime, your brain is kind of like "Ah-ha—I've got you to myself, with nothing else to distract us." So what does it do? It goes through all the things it is thinking about—fears, deep worries, regrets, dreams for the future . . . In REM sleep, the brain is processing, and processing, and processing. It's taking your experiences and deepest thoughts and attempting to work things out. Unfortunately, it isn't always successful—but it does ruin your deep sleep. Even worse, it spikes stress hormones like cortisol and epinephrine, which keep you awake and miserable. I experienced a few months of insomnia during a bout of anxiety, and boy, that was the worst experience of my life! There is nothing more miserable than being scared of another evening because you know you're going to toss and turn for hours. Let's discuss some solutions.

Should I Try Sleep Medications?

Sleep medications are widely prescribed by millions of primary care physicians and psychiatrists. In the United States, out of the sixty million people with sleep problems, almost thirteen million have taken sleep meds in the last thirty days. Women are three times more likely to use these drugs than men. It is also well known that the more educated you are, the more likely you are to use a sleeping pill. We learned in chapter 2 that it is typical for educated people to think so much that we talk ourselves out of sleep!

Should you use a sleep medication? As you know, I am a naturopathic physician. As a naturopath, I am certainly biased toward natural medicines. However, I am also trained to know that sometimes a conventional drug can help, especially in emergency situations. For example, if a patient had a life-threatening blood infection, and I knew an antibiotic could save them, but I was not sure that an herbal medicine would be effective, I would opt for the antibiotic in a second. A good doctor uses what is best for the patient at the time, especially when the benefit far exceeds the risk. But when it comes to sleep medications, in most cases, I do not believe there is greater benefit.

Most sleep medications are really *anxiety* medications. Sedative hypnotic drugs include Ambien, Xanax, Valium, and Lunesta. While the commercials for these drugs show happy people snug in bed with butterflies gently flying overhead, the medications are not as benign as the commercials make them look.

A study of thirty thousand people published in the February 2012 issue of the *British Medical Journal* found that when compared to those who did not take any sleep medications, people who took fewer than eighteen sleeping pills a year still had dramatically higher mortality rates. Higher doses were linked to a greater than 500 percent increase in death. The authors of this study concluded that sleep medications "may have been associated with 320,000 to 507,000 excess deaths in the USA alone." Like anxiety medications, sleeping pills are very addictive and can cause daytime dizziness, sleepiness, and poor motor skills—all symptoms you are trying to prevent. Because these drugs typically cause drowsiness, they do not support a healthy sleep architecture that allows you to get into the deep layers of slow wave sleep you need to feel refreshed. They take away the detoxifying and nourishing effects of sleep. So many of my patients who take Ambien say the same thing: "Well, I sleep, more or less, but I feel like I don't sleep at all." They feel hung over, and their anxiety slowly embeds itself in their minds.

You should know that the natural recommendations discussed below actually improve your sleep architecture in the long run. They promote "good" sleep—sleep the way nature intended, with all the health benefits.

So, to use medications or not to use them? I recommend this: if you are at a place where you really need sleep, and the natural supplements have not yet kicked in, then take what you need, but start to bring in the natural supports slowly and wean yourself off the drugs as soon as possible. In step 9, I will discuss how to safely use natural supports alongside conventional medications and eventually wean off for good.

Nine Steps to Improve Sleep

We have talked about what bad sleep is like, and we have discussed the pros and cons of sleep medications—now let's get to your real sleep solution. I have used versions of this plan with thousands of patients over ten years of clinical practice. In all that time, I have not met one patient who couldn't eventually sleep. You are not going to be the first.

I recommend the following steps to help get your sleep back on track.

Step 1: Go to Bed on Time

There's an old Chinese medicine proverb that says "one hour before midnight is worth two hours after midnight." While the ancient Chinese did not know about endocrinology (the study of hormones), this suggestion makes physiological sense. It encourages people to be in a still, dark place at a time when the onset of melatonin release allows for optimal sleep and circadian regulation.

Melatonin release starts around ten o'clock at night. Getting to bed at the right time optimizes its release. If you go to bed too much later, you will suppress melatonin and encourage stress hormone activity. This makes sense—the only animals that stay up past darkness are either running for their lives or hunting for food. Nocturnal animals like owls and fruit bats stay up at night and sleep during the day, but I suspect you are not related to them. Therefore, you should be sleeping at normal times. By staying up, you are releasing stress hormones and encouraging insomnia, delayed sleep phase syndrome, and early morning waking.

You may be saying to yourself, "Gosh, I go to bed at three or four in the morning; there's no way I can do eleven." That is totally okay. If you generally go bed at some point after midnight, and you are ready to make a positive change, I recommend backing up bedtime by fifteen minutes once a week, possibly to settle in at a ten thirty to eleven o'clock bedtime in the long run. If you are normally going to bed in the wee hours of the morning, it's great progress to get to bed by eleven thirty or midnight—for now. If you need to, you can use supplemental melatonin to help this process along. (Read more about melatonin in step 7.)

Step 2: Create Your Evening Ritual

Ritual and routine are crucial for healthy physiology. Animals need ritual. Children need ritual to feel secure. Adults need ritual to sleep. Creating an atmosphere in which your body and mind can expect the same thing, at the same time, while giving your body gentle signals of the slumber to come is vital to restore proper sleep.

Bright light tells the body "hey, it's daytime," and suppresses melatonin release. Dim your lighting during the evening hours. For your computer and devices, I recommend flux (*https://justgetflux.com*), a free, downloadable application that dims your computer/tablet and phone screens to a less melatonin-suppressing amber hue in the early evening.

Sipping a calming tea such as chamomile or lavender is a smart choice at this time. It is best to make a small cup and sip slowly—limit your liquid intake a few hours before bed so your bladder does not fill up and wake you during the night. As you create your own healthy sleep ritual, you will find comfort in consistency, and your body will learn to calm in preparation for sleep.

Step 3: Dim All the Lights Thirty Minutes Before Bed

Starting thirty minutes before bedtime, completely turn off anything with a bright light—computer, tablet, cell phone, television, and so on. Buy an orange light bulb (most lighting stores and large retailers carry these). Read calming literature under orange light—it will not suppress melatonin the way regular blue light can.

Step 4: Keep the Room Dark and Cool

Melatonin, human growth hormone, and other hormones are needed for repair and detoxification during sleep. When you sleep in a room that is too bright or too warm, these hormones are suppressed. How do you know if you are sleeping in a room with too much light? Try placing your hand one foot in front of your face. If you can see it, darken the room. Cover light sources, like cable boxes and clocks. Keep your cell phone charging in another room. Use completely occlusive blinds. Some of my patients get fancy and install automatic motors that open the blinds gradually in the morning to assure a slow introduction of light. But if you don't want to get too fancy, just uncover the window enough to allow a little morning light. Keep your room temperature around 68 degrees to ensure optimal melatonin secretion.

Step 5: Check In on Food and Blood Sugar

Occasionally, eating too late or having too much food in your stomach will raise your cortisol levels and make it hard for you to fall asleep. Some of my patients are also quite sensitive to certain foods and beverages (the most common are wine, spicy foods, dairy products, and fast food), which will keep them awake. If this happens to you, avoid these items after six p.m.

Alternately, having low blood sugar before bed can make it equally difficult to fall asleep. When blood sugar is low, the animal brain goes to hunt for food, and stress hormones are released. If your blood sugar is low, try eating protein and carbohydrates together (a little turkey with an apple slice or nut butter with a rice cracker) right before bed. But don't eat too much! Another trick I suggest to my patients is to keep a handful of blueberries near your bedside. If you wake up hungry, these can do the trick. If you are especially anxious and have nausea, prepare a cup of warm almond milk with cinnamon and keep it in a thermos. If you wake and feel nausea, you can calm your stomach with the warm beverage.

Step 6: Journal before Bed

Many of us lead hectic lives, and often we do not have even one quiet or relaxed moment during the day. Then you have to go to bed—even though you have been running full throttle. It is at bedtime, when we are alone, that the brain says, "Okay, now I've got you. Let's go over a few things." The brain (and your unconscious mind) wants to start processing things—lots of things, over and over and over. This is the moment when all the thoughts flood in at once: family issues, relationship worries, job stress, financial challenges, worries about nuclear war, and so on. These thoughts become overwhelming. They put you in stress mode, and your brain and body will not shut off.

In these cases, I strongly recommend a practice I use every evening: a few minutes before bed, I sit down under my orange light and make a "to-do list" for the next day. I write down the highest priorities and then fold the paper and put it aside, effectively "letting go" of my responsibilities until tomorrow. If you make this list, bring it to your psychologist or holistic practitioner—he or she will want to know what comes up during those nighttime hours. Walt Whitman said: "I do not think until I read what I write." While jotting them down may not fix the issues of concern, the very act of writing will help you to process them.

put anxiety behind you

Step 7: Natural Remedies for Sleep

I recommend that you start with the above steps for two weeks and see if your sleeping improves. If it does not balance out completely, then using natural medicines can be amazingly effective to finish the job.

Magnesium

Magnesium is one of my favorite supplements. It relaxes, is good for the heart and blood vessels, lowers inflammation in the body, and helps balance neurotransmitter production. Magnesium deficiency is common in people with mood problems. When there isn't enough magnesium around, your biological clock also suffers, which will disorganize your sleeping patterns.

Studies find that magnesium aids longer, better quality sleep, and less early morning waking. It will even help you fall asleep quicker. Magnesium is a one-stop shop when it comes to sleep.

Dosing is usually in the range of 400–500 mg a day. I often recommend 250 mg twice a day, with the last dose at bedtime. My favorite is the magnesium glycinate form; glycine is an amino acid known for its own calming effect. There is no known toxicity danger associated with magnesium, unless you have kidney problems. If you do, check with your doctor before taking magnesium. Also, some people's bowels are very sensitive, and magnesium may cause loose stools. If this happens to you, reduce the dose until your stomach feels better.

Melatonin

A powerful antioxidant, melatonin protects brain and nervous tissue. As a supplement, it was originally known as the best way to fix jet lag and is now known to help fight cancer due to its antioxidant properties and its ability to aid chemotherapy. Because studies have shown that low levels or delayed release of melatonin will cause anxiety, it is also popular as a sleep aid and antianxiety remedy. Some patients with anxiety might have worries about the safety of melatonin, but I assure you that it is quite safe and nonaddictive—it is even used as a sleep aid for children with attention deficit challenges.

Melatonin supplements are sold in various forms and dosages, from ½ mg up to 20 mg. While regular melatonin calms your body so it knows what time it should fall asleep, time-release formulas can help you stay asleep if you wake up during the night or early morning.

For trouble falling asleep, start with 1 mg of regular melatonin and dose up to 3 mg, taken forty-five minutes before bedtime. If you can fall asleep, but have trouble *staying* asleep, then use time-release melatonin (sometimes known as sustained release) in dosages starting at 3 mg and going up to 6 mg.

While melatonin has no toxicity in these doses, cut back a bit if you feel groggy in the morning. If you find that even 1 mg causes grogginess, then try liquid melatonin, which you can dose as little as $^1/_{10}$ mg. Some of my patients are that sensitive. The only time I would not use melatonin is if a person has nocturnal asthma or a cancer of the blood.

Several everyday foods contain small amounts of melatonin. Oats are known to have a calming effect on the body and do contain melatonin—but you would need to eat about twenty bowls of oats to ingest the amount of melatonin in a single pill. Montmorency cherries, ginger, tomatoes, bananas, and barley also contain minute amounts of melatonin. One study of tart cherry juice found a modest effect on sleep—cherries might be worth a try for mild insomnia issues.

Tryptophan

Tryptophan (sometimes referred to as L-tryptophan) is a naturally derived amino acid that serves as a precursor to the neurotransmitter serotonin, which is needed to help you stay asleep. Low levels of tryptophan contribute to generalized anxiety and panic attacks. Back in the early 1990s, a laboratory I was associated with at Yale University performed "tryptophan depletion studies" in which volunteers who were already prone to anxiety were put on a tryptophan-free diet. Within days, these people were extremely anxious, panicky, and unstable—and they had lots of trouble staying asleep.

I usually give people 500–1,000 mg of tryptophan at bedtime, but I may dose up to 2,500 mg. Take tryptophan at bedtime with a slice of simple carbohydrate (like an apple slice)—the carbohydrate will increase insulin levels, and insulin will promote tryptophan absorption in the brain. In my clinic, I use a supplement called Tryptophan Calmplete, which includes B vitamins. See appendix II for information on specific supplements.

Although most conventional psychiatrists are afraid to mix natural medicines like tryptophan with conventional medications, studies suggest that they can be safely combined. One eight-week randomized controlled trial of thirty patients with major depression combined 20 mg of Prozac (an SSRI medication) with 2,000 mg of tryptophan as daily treatment for major depressive disorder. This study demonstrated that combining tryptophan and an SSRI improved mood and helped patients stay asleep.

If you look up tryptophan on websites like WebMD, they are going to tell you tryptophan is unsafe. The reason for this is because in the early 1990s there was an incident of Eosinophilia Myalgia Syndrome, a condition contracted by thirty people who most unfortunately got sick (and some died) after ingesting tryptophan supplements. This tragic event occurred because the company making the supplement had no quality controls, and allowed the introduction of bacteria. These deaths had nothing to do with tryptophan itself. My sense is that the folks behind conventional websites like WebMD, who should be doing their homework, let these ideas persist on purpose. The drug companies who advertise with these websites then benefit from continuing the misinformation. I have taken tryptophan myself, have used it with family members and countless patients, with absolutely no problem, save for the side benefit of better sleep and mood.

Valerian
As an herbal sleep aid, valerian has been studied more than any other. The word's root, *valere,* is Latin for "good health." Despite popular understanding, you should know that valerian has absolutely no relationship with Valium—except for the fact that their names share the same first three letters.

Valerian is a great herb for you if you experience a strong anxiety component along with an inability to sleep. This herb boosts the calming gamma-aminobutyric acid (GABA) neurotransmitter, bringing down our "fight-or-flight" response.

In 2010, a research team looked at eighteen different medical trials of valerian that found it to be effective in treating anxiety and aiding sleep. For example, one trial found that about 530 mg of valerian, taken twice a day for four weeks, worked to help women's sleep quality over a placebo.

Typical dosage of valerian is 450 mg to 600 mg about two hours before bedtime. Patients with daily anxiety or needing more sleep support may add an equal dose in the late morning or early afternoon. In many cases, if valerian doesn't work for you right away, it may work best once you start taking it regularly. It has been shown to be safe in seniors and in children, but should not be used during pregnancy or breastfeeding. When patients are coming off anxiety medications, drug withdrawal can disrupt sleep. Valerian can also help with staying asleep when trying to wean off anxiety medications. In rat studies, valerian has been successfully used to help the animal wean off the benzodiazepine Valium.

To see if it would help in humans, a Brazilian research team in Sao Paulo tried the same with nineteen adults who had used benzodiazepines for an average of seven years at night to get to sleep. For fourteen days, they added either valerian at 100 mg three times a day or placebo pills. As the Valium was withdrawn, the patients taking that small amount of valerian had much better sleep quality and better withstood the side effects of drug discontinuation. At the end of the fourteen days, there was a significant decrease in nighttime waking in valerian subjects when compared to placebo subjects. The researchers concluded that there were no interactions between valerian and Valium, and valerian helped patients move through withdrawal symptoms, too. Since the active components of valerian may increase benzodiazepine activity, it is important to work with a knowledgeable practitioner if using valerian with benzodiazepine medications like Xanax or Valium.

Step 8: Get a Salivary Cortisol Test

For my patients with sleep issues, I always look at the patient's cortisol profile by checking saliva levels, as we will discuss in appendix I. If cortisol is too high at bedtime, during the night, or in the very early morning, I will consider adding supplemental phosphatidylserine or lactium at bedtime to lower cortisol levels, which can also help with sleep.

Step 9: Still Anxious?

If you still experience a lot of anxiety when going to bed, or if you are waking up in the middle of the night, try adding some supplemental GABA or phenibut to either take at bedtime or to use if you wake up at a certain time at night.

GABA and phenibut are used for plain old anxiety feelings. Either of these will help you get back to sleep if anxiety is keeping you up. First try the GABA in the range of 250 mg to 1,000 mg. If this doesn't work, you can try its stronger cousin phenibut, starting with 300 mg. More about GABA and phenibut in chapter 7.

Chinese Medicine for Sleep

We are going to talk about the benefits of acupuncture and Chinese medicine when we discuss mind-body therapies in chapter 6, but I will briefly cover Chinese medicine teachings in relation to sleep. There's a clock in Chinese medicine that associates time with the different organs in the body. Each organ represents a different time of the day and an emotion. In Chinese medicine theory, it is said that when you have a challenge that appears at a particular time every day, it is useful to consider which organ corresponds to that time, because each organ corresponds with an emotion that is often at the root of the challenge. While this may sound a bit far out to you, the Chinese have thousands of years of scientific observation to back up these associations. Here is a list that explains the organs and emotions associated with the early morning hours.

11:00 p.m. to 1:00 a.m.: Gallbladder—frustration, resentment, and pent-up anger

Treatment. Work on these emotions with your therapist or doctor and eat fiber-rich foods.

1:00 a.m. to 3:00 a.m.: Liver—stress and repressed emotion that is stuck in the body

Treatment. Work on these emotions, eat liver-healthy foods (such as kale, parsnips, artichoke, beets, and dandelion). Consider taking milk thistle supplement. Try a Chinese herb called "Free and Easy Wanderer," which helps gently move the liver energy.

3:00 a.m. to 5:00 a.m.: Lung—grief and great loss (like that of a loved one or pet), general worry

Treatment. Talk with your practitioner about these emotions while eating foods that are strengthening for the lungs, such as Asian pears. Also, avoid cold and raw foods, and focus on cooked foods, like stews and soups.

5:00 a.m. to 7:00 a.m.: Large intestine—grief, sadness, and worry.

Treatment. The large intestine is the organ of holding, so talk with your therapist or doctor about what you may be holding on to. Also, make sure you are getting plenty of fiber and consider taking glutamine powder (1 tsp per day) and a butyrate supplement, which helps the large intestine stay healthy.

Combining Supplements for Better Sleep

While any of the above supplements can be of value alone and get the job done, it is very common in holistic care to combine these natural remedies for even better results. For example, one double-blind study from Italy in 2011 gave people with sleeping challenges 5 mg of melatonin and 225 mg of magnesium to take about one hour before bedtime. Results showed significant improvements in sleep scores, and sleep quality improved. As can happen when you have enough sleep, the subjects felt more alert and "with it" the following day. Very often, I will start my patients on one supplement at a time, and then add others if the one supplement is not effective.

If you are worried about taking multiple supplements at one time, remember that supplements are not drugs. They are really more like foods in a capsule—foods that gently talk to your body and nudge it in the right direction. Sometimes you need to take a number of them to get the effect you are looking for.

Final Sleepy Note

I know we dove in to a good deal of information in this chapter. If you are having sleeping issues, it is worth trying multiple tactics. I know that when your sleep gets better, the anxiety will absolutely improve, too. Now that you have an idea of which supplements are the best, you can start to work with them. You may have to adjust timing and doses to fit your profile, but you can do it!

Checklist for Restorative Sleep

❏ Create sleep rituals

❏ Take supplements beneficial for sleep:

    ❏ Regular melatonin for falling asleep

    ❏ Time-release melatonin for staying asleep

    ❏ Magnesium for relaxation

    ❏ Tryptophan to help stay asleep

    ❏ Valerian for falling asleep

    ❏ GABA or phenibut to fall and stay asleep

❏ Check the Chinese clock and try Chinese herbs, foods, or therapy that correlate with the time you are waking up

4

exercise

Get comfortable with being uncomfortable.
—Jillian Michaels

Case: Mike with General Anxiety, Hypochondria, and Palpitations

Mike was a forty-seven-year-old financial analyst who lived outside of New York City and commuted almost two hours by car every day. He woke up at 4:30 a.m. in order to get to work by 7:00 a.m., and then worked until about 4:30 p.m. His evening commute was even more congested, and he returned home each night around 7:30 p.m. Mike was able to kiss his kids goodnight, eat a little something, and go to bed to do it all again the next day. He had been doing this for ten years.

He came to see me because over the last five years, he had experienced "heart flutters"—periods when his heart would race a mile a minute. He started worrying that he was gong to have a heart attack and was checked by some top cardiologists, who said the heart was fine. Once he knew his heart was not the problem, Mike started fretting about other aspects of his health. He worried that he might get colon cancer or that he would end up in an accident during his commute. These thoughts started taking over. Mike returned to his cardiologist, who told him that though his heart was fine, his blood pressure was up again. The doctor and gave him a blood pressure medication and recommended that Mike see a psychiatrist.

Because he didn't want drugs, Mike came to see me. Mike did have mild palpitations, and he told me about the constant thoughts of getting sick or injured. After listening closely to Mike's case, I recommended that he adjust his diet and eat more fiber, water, and vegetables. I also added a magnesium supplement for heart support.

A saliva stress test found that Mike's stress hormone levels were very high. I started him on some herbal ashwagandha, and, most importantly, emphasized the need for him to exercise, which would treat both the blood pressure and the anxiety. I explained to Mike that those stress hormones coursing through his body needed to be burnt off—and that in the wild, when an animal is stressed, it runs or fights, burning off those hormones. Mike just sits in his car! While his schedule was a tough one, Mike did set aside enough time to do a routine of weights, cardio, and boxing four times a week. Boxing and hitting the heavy bag is great when you need to burn stress hormones. In two months, Mike's weight was down, he was off his blood pressure medications, and was much happier—and he loved his new boxing hobby.

Hippocrates, who is regarded as the father of medicine, knew close to two thousand years ago that if someone had a mood problem, they needed to get up and move their body. He regarded outdoor exercise as the great mood balancer. Hippocrates knew how profoundly beneficial exercise was on mood, way before any researcher ever thought to measure exercise's positive impact on the brain.

Indeed, medical research has shown an amazing array of benefits on the body. Much of this you will already know, but here is just a partial list of what exercise can do.

- Lowers bad cholesterol and raises good cholesterol
- Prevents diabetes
- Prevents cancer
- Improves circulation
- Helps detoxification
- Lowers blood pressure
- Maintains weight and stops obesity
- Regenerates your mitochondria (the energy packs in your body)
- Extends life expectancy
- Prevents Alzheimer's and brain decline
- Stops depression
- And, of course, reduces anxiety

As Phil Rizzuto, former ball player and announcer for the New York Yankees used to say: "Ho-leee cowwwww!" Yes, holy cow indeed. What drug or supplement does all that? None that I know of, or I would be taking it for sure!

For me, exercise is key to staying anxiety-free. I find it gets me out of negative patterns before they really start and take hold. For instance, sometimes I'll be talking a bit fast, breathing shallowly, or saying something negative to my wife. Because she knows me well, she will stop the conversation, look at me, and say, "You know what? You should go for a run, and then come back and talk to me."

Experts believe that exercise may be the most effective "drug" of all time for both anxiety and depression. Exercise has been shown to bring down anxiety, minimize panic attacks, and slash negative mood, while simultaneously improving self-esteem and even memory. There is also a great body of research that shows how exercise may be the best antidepressant of all time, too.

I know that sometimes when you are anxious, the feeling of your heart beating hard and fast can feel like an actual anxiety attack. As Jillian Michaels reminds us, we should get used to this type of healthy discomfort. Acclimating to exercise as part of your anxiety plan will help you work through this issue.

How Does Exercise Help Anxiety?

So how does exercise help keep you less anxious? There are a few mechanisms involved.

In chapter 2, we discussed the idea that thoughts and fears drive the middle part of the brain and agitate the body. That feeling is called the fight-or-flight response. It is the "I am anxious because I need to run from a bear right now" feeling. If you need to run from a bear in real life, what do you do? You run from that bear—and run you should. Your body makes stress hormones like epinephrine and cortisol, and as you run, you burn up those stress hormones. In that case, anxiety is a good thing—it saves you from getting eaten! And when it's over, your stress hormones are all used up, so you feel calm and relaxed.

Of course, in modern life, physically running away is rarely an option. Let's say you are not in the forest, facing a bear. Instead, you are at work, in a board meeting, and you start to have those familiar anxious feelings. If you ran away at that moment, you might not have a job when you got back. So you sit there, and you get more panicky. Those stress hormones course through your body and make you feel anxious (heart palpitations, sweating, depersonalization and floaty feeling, stomach pain . . .). You're trapped—you have no opportunity to burn them off, but still you are feeling their effects.

Regular exercise stops the trapped feeling by lowering the overall level of stress hormones. People who exercise regularly find that, even if they get stressed out in that board meeting, the feelings do not overwhelm them.

There are a few physiological effects at play when it comes to the mood benefits of regular exercise. Besides burning those stress hormones, exercise also protects the brain areas needed for stable mood.

Exercise also increases the production of an important central nervous system molecule called brain-derived neurotrophic factor (BDNF). BDNF plays a strong role in building nerve cells (called neurogenesis), and it helps the nervous system repair damage. Just as building and repair are needed to keep a house in good shape, these building and repair functions are critical for keeping your brain and mood in shape.

Exercise has also been shown to maintain the brain's hippocampus. The hippocampus is an area vital to mood, spatial relationships, and memory. A study of 120 older adults with dementia showed that after one year of moderate-intensity aerobic exercise three days a week, subjects actually increased their hippocampal volume by about 2 percent. Since 2 percent is around the amount expected for an older adult to lose per year with natural aging, the study showed that exercise effectively reverses age-related loss in brain volume. The group that did not do aerobic exercise, but instead only stretching and toning work, experienced the normal 2 percent decrease in hippocampal volume over that year.

Research Evidence for Exercise and Anxiety

Compared to leading antidepressant and antianxiety medications, exercise is shown to be quite effective. One randomized controlled trial (RCT) of 156 adults compared exercise to the antidepressant Zoloft. Researchers learned that the effects of exercise took a little longer to kick in, but the exercise worked just as well as the drug in the long run and showed significantly lower relapse rates (8 percent versus 31 percent) than subjects in the medication group. A second RCT looked at patients of at least fifty years of age who experienced depression. Researchers recommended that one group of volunteers start a course of exercise, and the other take antidepressant medications. Again, there was quicker improvement in the drug group, but after sixteen weeks, the exercise caught up with equal benefits.

Exercise has clear benefits for anxiety states as well. We talked earlier about how the flood of the stress hormone cortisol beats up the brain—especially the area called the hippocampus, which will shrink down when it is exposed to too much stress hormone. Animal studies have demonstrated how exercise can actually reverse this shrinkage.

As we discussed above, human studies show the same benefit. Exercise helps create new brain cells, and can help calm them when they are overexcited. Recent mouse studies at Princeton University suggest that those animals that exercise not only grow new nerve cells but also create more that are able to release calming neurotransmitters, especially GABA.

Exercise also helps detoxify your body. Detoxification is necessary to clear the brain and nervous system of inflammation—and inflammation causes anxiety. This may be one of the many reasons that exercise helps anxiety—by calming an inflamed brain.

Exercise's ability to increase circulation brings more blood flow through the liver, lungs, and kidneys, your main organs of detox.

Exercise helps remove unwanted subcutaneous fat—these are the fat cells that hold many unwanted toxins in storage. Exercise also moves flow through the lymphatic system. The lymph system is basically the drainage system for the body—it collects waste products and toxins. While the cardiovascular system has a heart to pump the blood around, the lymphatic system has no such built-in pump. But every time you move a muscle, your lymphatic system gets a chance to move its contents into the veins, which helps expel the waste. The lymph system dumps the inflammatory garbage from your body's metabolic processes. When the muscles do not move, the body cannot detox, and inflammation takes over. Finally, exercise forces the body to take in good, deep breaths and assures better cell oxygenation.

"Hey, Doc—I Don't Know about You, But I Don't Sweat"

If you don't exercise, you will also miss out on sweat—a prime method your body uses to clean out and detoxify. Many patients tell me "well, I don't really sweat." This may be true if you are a canine—dogs do not have sweat glands and must pant and keep their mouth open to regulate their temperature. There are a few exceedingly rare medical conditions where a person does not actually have sweat glands—I doubt you have one of those. Other than that, you should be sweating it out like the rest of us. If you exercise and still believe you do not sweat, you may not be exercising hard enough—or you might be dehydrated, so your body is conserving water.

The truth is, many of us do not sweat enough. Only three in ten adults get the recommended amount of physical activity. We live and work in temperature-controlled environments all day, then ride in trains, cars, and buses with more air conditioning. Typically, we don't sweat because we are not given the chance. There are very few methods humans can use to get rid of chemicals from the body: defecation, urination, exhalation, and sweating it out. Human sweat glands help regulate temperature by bringing warm moisture to the surface of the skin, which causes cooling as the water evaporates. But their secondary role as detoxifier is not a minor one. Known as the "third kidney," your skin has over 2.6 million tiny pores that can help clear as much as 30 percent of bodily wastes through perspiration. Sweat is mostly water, but also contains urea (a breakdown product of proteins from the kidneys) and trace metals and minerals. Mercury is one of the many toxins known to be flushed out via sweat.

To help get your sweating going, start an exercise routine. If you already work out but you are not sweating with the routine you have, consider increasing the intensity of your workout (unless your doctor says otherwise). Increasing intensity could mean increasing your pace or the angle of incline on your cardio machine. Sometimes, working with a trainer will help you safely find inspiration for perspiration. Often, people do not like to feel uncomfortable— and getting to the point of sweating might feel uncomfortable. If you have anxiety, just know those feelings of discomfort are normal. You know that exercise can't hurt you—and in reality, it will help you a lot.

Yoga enthusiasts may try bikram yoga, a yoga practiced in a 105-degree temperature for ninety minutes. Outside your exercise habit, you may also want to consider adding a steam sauna for increased detoxification. Hot and wet steam saunas are more effective than dry saunas. Steam saunas create beads of moisture, which adhere and coat the skin almost instantaneously. These prevent the body from losing heat through the process of evaporation. This may accelerate the detoxification and healing processes, which take place within the body when body temperature rises. More studies on this are needed.

Don't know where to start? Try this simple detox exercise protocol.

♦ Beginners: thirty minutes of gentle interval aerobic activity four days a week, and two days a week of yoga detoxification poses

♦ Intermediate and advanced: one hour of cardio, add intervals to the last thirty minutes, four days a week (see *www.drpeterbongiorno.com/interval* for interval training directions), plus two days of resistance work followed by detoxification yoga

Exercise Instead of Sleep?

Animal studies also teach us that if an animal is exhausted and hasn't slept enough, the benefits of exercise do not seem to hold. So, it's super important that you create a strong sleep schedule first and not dip into needed sleep time in order to exercise. Do not trade sleep to get in your exercise.

How to Get Started with Exercise

If you are new to exercise, I generally recommend starting nice and slow. Pick something you enjoy. I love being outside as much as possible, so running works well for me. I also go to the gym a few days a week to do resistance and strength training, because running alone doesn't build muscle the way we need for long-term health.

When you are first starting out, it is very important to go easy in order to avoid injury. Get outside in nature if possible, in green areas among the trees and in the sunlight. Jogging, walking, and tai chi are all wonderful. If you have any limitations with weight bearing or movement, then think about swimming or getting an elliptical training machine instead, for these exercises are gentler. A few of my patients who can't walk or move their legs use a tabletop arm pedal exerciser.

Earlier, we discussed an amazing study that showed that you can actually grow a part of the brain called the hippocampus with exercise. This part of the brain naturally shrinks with age, and anxiety accelerates this shrinkage even more. But according to the study, you have the power to reverse these processes with exercise. If you would like to replicate one of the hippocampus-building studies, it is broken down below.

Hippocampal Growth Exercise

Four out of seven days:

- Low-intensity warm-up on a treadmill or stationary bicycle for five minutes
- Stretching for five minutes
- Aerobic training for forty minutes: choose among stationary bike, treadmill running, StairMaster climbing, or training on an elliptical machine
- Cool down and stretching for ten minutes

Checklist for Exercise

- ❏ Create a schedule for at least three or four days a week and start as gently as needed
- ❏ Work up to five or six days a week, using alternating cardio and weight training
- ❏ When comfortable, bring in interval work to your cardio training

5

guts, food, and blood sugar

Unquiet meals make ill digestions.
Thereof the raging fire of fever bred,
And what's a fever but a fit of madness?

—Shakespeare

Case: Sarah with Stomach Issues and Anxiety

Forty-nine-year-old Sarah came to me with anxiety, sleeping problems, and hot flashes. The hot flashes had started about ten months before, and the sleep and anxiety issues had been ongoing for six months. She had been to a few doctors already, both conventional and holistic. Her conventional doctors said, "This is hormonal—this happens with perimenopause and you may have to ride it out." To help her ride it out, she was prescribed Xanax for daytime anxiety and Ambien for sleeping. While the Xanax did calm her down, she felt the Ambien gave her "a weird sleep . . . almost like I didn't sleep." Unhappy with the medication route overall, Sarah tried a holistic doctor, who recommended bio-identical hormones. Because Sarah's mom had breast cancer, she did not want to try these.

Sarah explained that the anxiety was getting worse without the Xanax, but there were no other options. In our first visit, I asked her about her digestion: she said it was okay. Prodding further, I learned it wasn't okay at all. She had bowel movements two or three times a week at the most. Occasionally, she wouldn't have a bowel movement for almost a week, and then have a big bowel movement followed by diarrhea. I asked her if she had ever been diagnosed with Irritable Bowel Syndrome (IBS). She told me that she was diagnosed with IBS in her late teens, but "it wasn't that bad, and I learned to deal with it." It turned out that she had some traumatic experiences in her early teens, and that up to this day, had a fair amount of repressed anxiety that finally came out with the hormonal changes.

I explained to Sarah that digestion is key to neurotransmitter balance and emotions. Stress and repressed emotions will shut down digestion—so both of them need to be worked on together. While a hormonal change might have spurred on Sarah's symptoms, my sense was that the hormonal change was merely the straw that broke the camel's back.

Sarah started getting counseling to deal with her repressed emotions. We worked on her digestion by adding more high-fiber foods (green vegetables, flax meals, and some fruit) and having her eat small meals a few times a day. We added a little psyllium fiber twice a day, and an enteric coated peppermint oil to help her colon movement. For sleep, I started Sarah on time-release melatonin and had her work on the sleeping rituals discussed in chapter 3. Finally, I recommended soy foods to go along with her flax meal and help balance estrogen fluctuations.

Within three weeks, Sarah's anxiety calmed and her sleep improved. She started having bowel movements every day. This is a fine example of the benefits of working on digestion first, to allow the body to rebalance and calm down.

The Anxiety-Gut Connection

How often have you heard about the intimate connection between your feelings and your digestive tract? Probably more times than you can count. If you don't know what I am talking about, think about whether you have ever heard these phrases:

"It's a gut feeling."
"There are butterflies in my stomach."
"The way to a man's heart is through his stomach."
"My heart is in my stomach."

Research also bears this out: a 2008 Roman study looked at 1,641 people with gastrointestinal problems and found that the vast majority had anxiety and about one quarter also suffered depression. Despite these clear associations, modern psychiatry has still all but ignored the ironclad link between the gastrointestinal system and anxiety. This is one reason why I think the current mode of modern psychiatry will never be able to fully treat mood disorder.

Naturopathic doctors have an old saying: "If you don't know what is wrong or what to treat, then treat the gut." Digestion is the go-to system for difficult-to-treat cases. For hundreds of years, holistic practitioners have known that improved digestion leads to better overall health, including mood. Modern science is starting to catch up to this concept.

Conventional medicine has relegated all mood disorders to the realm of the psychiatrist. Appendix I runs down a list of blood tests that crosses over into the territory of the hematologist (who looks at red and white blood cells), endocrinologist (who looks at hormonal balance), neurologist (who looks at the nervous system), cardiologist (who looks at the heart and blood vessels), toxicologist (who is concerned with toxins in the body), and nutritionist (who thinks about levels of vitamins in the body). That is a dream team of people covering many more bases than just the realm of psychiatry. In this chapter, I will discuss why the gastroenterologist (stomach and digestion doctor) should be getting involved, too.

Michael Gershon's book, *The Second Brain*, took a new perspective on the digestive system. Gershon argued that digestion is not just about sucking in nutrition from food and pooping out what is not needed; the digestive system also affects the brain and nervous system. Gershon explained to the public, for the first time, that the digestive tract has a robust nervous and hormonal system that is as active and effective as the actual central nervous and hormone systems themselves. Sometimes called the "enteric" nervous system (the word "enteric" refers to the digestive tract), the gastrointestinal tract is a major source of neurotransmitters in the body and is closely related to anxiety and mood.

The digestive tract breaks down protein (from foods like meat and nuts) into the component amino acid tryptophan. In the digestive tract, tryptophan is transformed into the neurotransmitter serotonin. When your digestion isn't working well (often due to stress, poor diet, sleep problems, and toxins), there is a lot more inflammation in the digestive tract. And when inflammation is high, the body is much less prepared to absorb tryptophan into the brain.

A prime example of this is in patients who have celiac disease, where chronic inflammation leads to poor nutrient absorption. Additionally, irritating foods and inflammation will spur the digestive tract to send high amounts of serotonin into the digestive system as a protective mechanism, where it encourages fast movement as a means to empty out the gut. Did you ever get frightened and later on end up with diarrhea? This action of serotonin is a prime cause of diarrhea in people who have mood disorders, poor diet, and high stress.

The scientific research clearly shows how bowel problems are correlated with mood. About 20 percent of patients with functional bowel disorders such as irritable bowel syndrome have diagnosable psychiatric illness. Almost a third of patients with major depression are thought to have constipation, and patients with irritable bowel syndrome are prone to both anxiety disorders and depression. In my experience with patients, I often find that people with anxiety previously had a digestive problem for years, or even decades, before.

How many people do you know who have self-esteem challenges? Women are especially prone to suffer from low sense of self. Are you one of them? Interestingly, bowel movements are intimately linked with a woman's sense of self-worth and her ability to maintain a relationship.

An interesting study published in the journal *Gut* followed thirty-four women, aged between nineteen and forty-five years, who had suffered significant constipation for at least five years. Compared to women who did not have any constipation, the constipated group had poorer health, difficulty forming close relationships, and described themselves as "less feminine." The constipated group also experienced reduced flow of blood to the rectum; this low rectal blood flow was strongly associated with both anxiety and depression.

It was also correlated with negative body symptoms and difficulty socializing. The authors of the study concluded that a woman's individual psychological makeup alters the function of the nerves that link the brain to the digestive tract. When a woman is stressed, gut function slows down, resulting in constipation. Since it is known that most neurotransmitters needed for healthy mood are made in the digestive tract, it makes sense that slowed gut function will impact how a women feels about herself, and how she responds in a relationship.

How to Avoid Constipation

Now you know the reason why good moods need good bowel function. It makes sense to help get the pipes moving. I recommend that patients move their bowels at least one time a day (preferably in the morning). Though some medical texts cite three times a week as "normal," now you know better. Steps to create your healthiest bowel movements include:

1. **Drink water.** Besides helping absorption of important amino acids like tryptophan, water keeps things flowing through the body. If you don't have enough water, the body will steal it from the colon, making the feces dry out and causing constipation. Sipped throughout the day, two liters (about sixty-four ounces) of pure, clean water is ideal for most people.

2. **Adequate fiber intake.** About twenty-five grams a day will go a long way for your best mood. You will find fiber in plenty of fruits and vegetables, as well as flax meal, psyllium, or organic dried prunes. Studies show that about seven grams (a little over a teaspoon) of psyllium twice a day in a big glass of water works best to help senior patients wean off addictive laxative supplements.

3. **Stress reduction work.** Do you poop better when you are on vacation? Many of my patients tell me that when they are relaxed, they move their bowels every day, but when they are home and going to work, things shut down. This suggests that stress is a major factor in their digestive process. Whether it is acupuncture, meditation, yoga, or taking a vacation, regular stress reduction is important. We will discuss stress reduction techniques in the next chapter.

4. **Natural laxatives.** If the above is not enough, then natural supplements will come to the rescue. Magnesium supplements are gentle and can help the bowels move quicker—typical doses for laxative effect start at 400 mg and may move up to 1,000 mg. Magnesium oxide is the cheapest form of magnesium. While I don't recommend it for anxiety, the oxide version has the best

stool softening effect. Also, concentrated Epsom salt baths have a laxative effect—Epsom salts are made from magnesium sulphate and support absorption through the mucosa in the anal area. High doses of vitamin C (three or more grams a day) can also act to loosen stool.

In extreme cases, I recommend laxative herbs like senna or cascara, which can be taken as a tea. Stronger pill forms can also help. I do think these herbs should be used sparingly and only in the short term (a few days, up to a week or two) while you are bringing in the methods discussed earlier. Any laxative can create a situation where the body becomes dependent on it. Over time it stops working, leaving you even more constipated than before. Laxatives are only a short-term solution and do not fix the root cause of the constipation.

Steps to a Healthy Digestive Tract

Now that you understand the connection between digestion and anxiety, it is time we put a plan in place to work on creating your healthy digestive tract.

1. **Fix constipation.** If you are not having regular bowel movements, then review the above steps as the first order of business to achieving healthful digestion.

2. **Before-meal ritual: breathing and bitters.** A deep diaphragmatic breath or two before a meal will help you calm your body and return circulation to your digestive tract. Also, a little aperitif before a meal is relaxing and will help spur enzyme production. Aperitifs (also called "digestifs" when used after meals) are small drinks that typically contain alcohol and bitter herbs like gentian. These bitter herbs increase digestive enzyme production and stimulate bile in order to help prepare for protein and fat digestion. If you are avoiding alcohol, you can add bitters like gentian and skullcap extract to warm water or seltzer instead.

3. **Chewing, chew, chew.** There's an old saying: "Nature castigates those who don't masticate." The teeth are the hardest substance in your body. You need them to pulverize your food. Birds guzzle their food whole, but they have gizzards—stomachs with teeth in them made for grinding—and you do not. So you have to chew your food well.

   If you do not chew and chew well, even healthy foods will be more likely to spur inflammatory reactions in your body. Poorly broken down food particles will stimulate the gut immune system, which comprises about 70 percent of your total immune system, creating inflammation throughout the body. Also, lack of chewing means less digestion of carbohydrates—many patients with bowel disorders like Crohn's disease, ulcerative colitis, and small intestinal bowel over-growth will improve if carbohydrates were broken down properly in the mouth as nature intended.

About fifty years ago, in the era of *Leave to Beaver,* Americans chewed their food as many as twenty-five times before swallowing. Current reports state that Americans chew only ten times at most. I believe most people do not even chew that many times. I know that if I do not think about it, I tend to chew things once or twice, and swallow my food virtually whole. Take a poop test: next time you have a bowel movement, look at your poop to see if there is food that looks like it did before you put it in your mouth. If there is, you are definitely not chewing it enough.

The next time you eat, remember to take a deep relaxing breath before starting. Then take reasonable-sized bites and count: chew the food twenty times until it is texturally unrecognizable.

4. **Choose healthy foods.** Generally, eating whole foods as prescribed by the Mediterranean diet (see Food for Your Best Mood section below) is a great place to start. If your digestion is not strong enough yet, soups and foods cooked in the slow cooker may be easiest for the digestive tract to break down and assimilate. Check out my website, *www.drpeterbongiorno.com/slowcook,* for my favorite anxiety-lowering slow cooker recipes.

5. **Relaxation and psychological work.** For your gut to be robust, you need to be as calm as possible. When the animal thinks a bear is going to attack him, the primitive brain shunts all energy to the organs needed to fight or run (muscles, brain, heart). This is called the sympathetic response. Part of this sympathetic response is shutting down the organ systems that are not needed. You guessed it—the digestive tract gets shut down, for there is no eating when you are running from a bear. (By the way, you can forget about the libido, too, for there will be no interest in sex while running from a bear either—which explains why anxiety lowers fertility.) Once the bear is no longer a threat, the animal returns to parasympathetic response, also known as "rest and digest." Now, digestion can resume.

Chapter 6's discussion on breathing, meditation, acupuncture, and massage can help you to lower stress hormones and return to the parasympathetic mode. Working on your thoughts, as we talked about in chapter 2, will be invaluable as well.

Food for Your Best Mood

If you bring a dog to the veterinarian for virtually any health issue, the first thing the vet will ask is: "What do you feed this dog?" This is because the vet is trained to know that what the animal ingests will affect its health considerably, and a good first place to look when health is sub-optimal is the diet.

Although a tenet still virtually ignored by most of modern medicine, it stands to reason that what you eat is going to affect your body in a substantial way. Poor diet will increase the likelihood a disease, especially if you are already predisposed. On the other side of the coin, eating healthy foods leads to better health. In this section, we will discuss the benefits of good nutrition, and then identify some specific food choices particularly appropriate for anxiety.

More and more studies are showing how healthy food can help prevent anxiety and block the bodily harm that occurs with mental illness. But which is the best diet? I would like to share with you a personal story. Despite the fact that medical school should be a place to learn about health, I spent my first year of medical school at the naturopathic program at Bastyr University in Seattle as a stressed-out student trying to do my best with a volume of information that appeared beyond my capacity (at least my negative thoughts were telling me so). While I had done a lot of psychological work to beat anxiety in my twenties, now that I was in my thirties, a second round of anxiety was approaching, due in part to the choices I was making.

During that year, I accumulated more and more study hours at the expense of exercise and sleep. There was lots of reading and memorizing, and I ate mostly quick foods, usually in the form of carbohydrates to feed a brain that was looking for sugar (those homemade human head-sized cafeteria chocolate chip cookies didn't help me make better decisions either). It is interesting—the brain makes up about 2 percent of the mass in our body, but it burns through about half of the body's total calories. This is why frenetic students and stressed out people in general love to eat cookies, bagels, and cakes. Ironically, while I was studying health, I was becoming less healthy. By my second year, I had terrific insomnia, anxiety, regular bouts of racing heartbeat, and irritable mood. And my mood gradually declined as the months of insomnia continued.

My parents, both of whom emigrated to the United States from Sicily before I was born, booked a trip to Italy for early summer. Knowing I was not feeling well, they asked me to join them. My mother said, "You will feel better—you should come." I was feeling so awful that the thought of taking a trip to Sicily and being five thousand miles away from my Seattle home sounded like too much. I wasn't sleeping as it was—I was sure a few time zone changes would really mess me up. But Italian mother guilt got to me, and I agreed to go.

After a six-hour trip from Seattle to New York, then a six-hour flight to Rome and a one-and-a-half-hour connecting flight to Palermo, I landed in the small airport and was greeted by arid Palermo sun. I met my parents in Sicily near the coastal hometown of my father, Castellemare del Golfo. Worried about me, my mother did what any loving Italian mother would and cooked me a meal. This one was Sicilian olive oil, fresh fish bought in town a few hours prior, locally grown vegetables, a small slice of fresh artisan bread, and a little wine. The fish there is sold so fresh, it is not even kept on ice— it is caught in the waters nearby, wrapped in seaweed, and sold hours later. After I ate, I did what any Sicilian man would do: I took a nap in the Sicilian sun.

By the next day, I was sleeping like a baby and my anxiety and physical symptoms had vanished! Now, this was not a double-blind, placebo-controlled study, but when I look back now, I wonder if all I needed was some good Mediterranean sun and food—the kind of food that kept my ancestors healthy, the kind of food Hippocrates gave to his patients.

Getting away from the books and the tests helped, too. Think about it: I had been slogging through the dark grey Seattle days, taking test after test, for a whole year. I had not seen the sun (which means I wasn't getting much vitamin D either). As I mentioned, my food intake was high in carbohydrates. When I had the opportunity to soak in the sun, healthy oils, fresh fish fatty acids, and vibrant green nutrients, it was like telling my body: "Don't worry, you are going to be all right."

Part of my healing was the Mediterranean diet's ability to talk to my body. And it's not just me it talks to—the diet has been well studied in many other people. One landmark five-year study out of Spain looked at the lives and eating patterns of ten thousand people and found that those who followed the Mediterranean diet were 50 percent less likely to develop anxiety or depression. The study found that specifically, intake of fruits, nuts, beans, and olive oil supported mood best.

The Mediterranean diet isn't just good for your brain; it's good for your body, too. Other studies have shown that the inner linings of the blood vessels (called the endothelial linings) were much healthier in people who ate a Mediterranean diet. When those vessels are in good shape, the chances of getting cardiovascular disease are much lower. Even more, studies by the same group found that people who ate in this healthy way also had higher levels of brain-derived neurotrophic factor (BDNF). We have talked about this molecule a few times already—it's secreted by the nervous system and is critical for growth, repair, and survival of healthy brain and nervous system cells. BDNF has been shown to be low in people with anxiety.

Components of a Mediterranean Diet to Add to Yours

◆ High amounts of monounsaturated fats (fish oil, olive oils, flax oil) and low amounts of saturated fats

◆ High intake of legumes (beans)

◆ High fish intake (stick to low-mercury fish)

◆ Intake of whole grain cereals and breads (add these unless gluten intolerant)

◆ High intake of fruits (high-antioxidant berries are at the top of the list)

◆ High intake of raw nuts (1/2 cup a day)

◆ High intake of vegetables (can't eat too many of these)

◆ Moderate alcohol intake (one small glass a day at most—do not add if alcoholism or liver issues are a concern)

◆ Moderate intake of milk and dairy products (unless sensitive to cow's milk)

◆ Low intake of meat and meat products (and keep these grass-fed and organic)

One of the head researchers of this wonderful food research, Dr. Miguel Angel Martinez-Gonzalez, offered his understanding of the advantages of the Mediterranean diet:

> The membranes of our neurons (nerve cells) are composed of fat, so the quality of fat that you are eating definitely has an influence on the quality of the neuron membranes, and the body's synthesis of neurotransmitters is dependent on the vitamins you're eating.

It is clear that Dr. Martinez-Gonzalez gets it: the food you eat and the vitamins you take in affect how your nervous system is built, which affects your neurotransmitter levels, which affect your emotional state.

A recent study from the *Canadian Journal of Psychiatry* looked closely at the foods and nutrient intakes of ninety-seven people with confirmed mood disorders. Researchers considered intake of fats, carbohydrates, and proteins, as well as vitamins and minerals. They found clear correlations between mental health function and diet. Intake of linoleic acid (an omega-6 fatty acid, which we will discuss later on), riboflavin, niacin, folic acid, vitamins B6 and B12, pantothenic acid, calcium, phosphorus, potassium, and iron, as well as magnesium and zinc, all played roles. When dietary supplement use was added to the nutrient intakes from food, mental health scores did even better, suggesting that supplementation, along with healthy foods, can play a role in helping anxiety disorder.

Often, my patients and fellow practitioners will ask me which, in my opinion, is the best diet. While I think this question is best answered on a patient-by-patient basis, if I did not know the individual or her health history, I would recommend the Mediterranean diet. Although no one diet is completely perfect for every individual due to possible allergies and sensitivities, there is reason to believe that the benefits of the Mediterranean diet may far surpass other diets for anyone with mood problems. Again, while no one diet is 100 percent effective and healthy for every person, the Mediterranean diet is considered one of the most healthful for many different people and conditions, and the research seems to support this bold statement.

Some Specifically Healthy Foods

We have talked about a system of eating called the Mediterranean diet. Now, let's break down food a little further in regards to how it can affect, and help, your mood.

Protein Sources

The Centers for Disease Control suggests that at least one third of the US population is obese. But believe it or not, despite all this overeating, many people are actually still undernourished and not getting enough protein. Americans tend to eat lots of high-carbohydrate foods (breads, bagels, muffins, cakes, rice). These foods have little to no quality protein. Low protein intake is especially a problem for people inclined to have anxiety issues for two reasons. One is that proteins break down to amino acids, which are the building blocks of our molecules of emotion, the neurotransmitters. And second, it is very challenging to regulate blood sugar with insufficient protein—and blood sugar dysregulation is associated with anxiety. Pregnant women who eat a vegetarian diet typically low in protein have a 25 percent greater likelihood for high levels of anxiety symptoms, likely due to low protein levels. So, how much protein should you be getting? To help understand how much protein a person generally needs, use the formula below:

$$\left(\text{weight in pounds} \div 2.2\right) \times 0.8 = \text{grams of protein you need per day}$$

For example, a 120-pound person will require about 44 grams of protein. Please note that elite athletes should multiply by 1.2 grams instead of 0.8 grams. Also important to note is that excess protein can also be a problem. Way too much protein (say, 150 grams or more) can actually suppress central nervous system serotonin levels, which will negatively affect mood. Also, remember that anyone with kidney disease may need to decrease his or her intake below the above formula recommendation.

The healthiest protein sources are beans, raw nuts and seeds, tofu, fish, natural poultry, and grass-fed meats.

Fish and Healthy Oils

There is ample evidence showing that people who eat less seafood have higher rates of mood disorder. Conversely, solid research also tells us that higher intake of fish may help prevent and treat these disorders.

Seafood intake is shown to lower both anxiety and depression. One study showed that those who rarely or never ate dark and oily fish were 43 percent more likely to suffer from anxiety, in comparison to those who ate it one to three times a week or more. One thorough review spanning thirteen countries demonstrated an inverse relationship between intake of fish and poor mood, whether it is anxiety or depression.

There are two main types of healthy omega-3 fatty acids in fish: eicosapentanoic acid (EPA) and docosahexaenoic acid (DHA). It is believed these substances help balance inflammation in the body and brain, and lower the likelihood of anxiety. These omega-3 fats are especially high in wild salmon, striped bass, mackerel, rainbow trout, halibut, and sardines. While science is still trying to understand whether EPA or DHA is more important, it is clear that individuals with anxiety and depression who eat less fish show marked depletions in omega-3 fatty acids in blood cell fats compared to people who do not have these mood disorders.

The standard American diet (with the very appropriate acronym, "SAD") tends to be quite low in healthy omega-3 fish oil and high in omega-6 oils. Omega-6 oils are found in saturated fats and red meats. We already know that diets with high omega-6 to omega-3 ratios increase the risk of heart disease and contribute to mood problems. Swedish researchers who studied seniors found that both bad mood and markers of inflammation increased with higher omega-6 to omega-3 fatty acid ratios. Too much saturated fat heightens inflammation and anxiety even further. Please note that I am not suggesting that a person eat no saturated fat—a little is good, too (maybe 15 to 20 grams a day), but too much will weigh down your brain.

Since the brain and nervous system are made of mostly fat and water, it stands to reason that healthy dietary fats (and plenty of good clean water) are crucial for your best mood. While we have focused mostly on omega-3 fats, other healthy oils, such as cold-pressed extra virgin olive oil (which contains brain-supportive omega-9 fats or oleic acids) and flax oil are also highly recommended. Look for organic and natural food sources of these oils—they contain lower levels of pesticides, neurotoxins, and metals. And since our waters are pretty contaminated with mood-altering toxins, please be aware of the fish you include in your diet—be sure to keep the mercury content low.

Here's a list from the National Resource Defense Council for identifying low-mercury fish:

Low mercury, okay to eat 2–3 times a week:	
• Anchovies	• Sardines
• Catfish	• Scallops
• Flounder	• Shrimp
• Herring	• Sole
• Rainbow trout	• Tilapia
• Salmon	

Moderate mercury, eat once or twice a month:
• Cod
• Snapper

High mercury, try to avoid or eat rarely:
• Halibut
• Lobster
• Mackerel
• Sea bass
• Tuna

Probiotic Foods and the Microbiome
In recent years, researchers have uncovered amazing new information about the role of the microbiome, the main resident of your digestive tract lining. The microbiome includes all the microorganisms that inhabitant our digestive tract—about 100 trillion bacteria. The microbiome is a key player in the two-way communication between the digestive tract and the brain. As you have learned, digestion is an important player in best mood, and a healthy bacterial balance in the microbiome is an important part of healthy digestion. Probiotic foods not only help digestion but are also key factors in obesity, hormonal balance, healthy kidney function, and much more.

Medical research is uncovering just how these little critters really work to help us feel our best. These healthy germs boost mood in two important ways: they generate the neurotransmitter GABA, and they enhance the docking stations (called receptors) for GABA as well. As we have seen, GABA is an amino acid known to calm overactive areas of the brain.

Animal studies showed that when mice consume probiotics, they are generally more "chilled out" than the control mice. The mice that ate probiotics also had lower levels of corticosterone, the mouse version of the human stress hormone cortisol, in response to stress.

So probiotics work to lessen anxiety in mice—but you are not a mouse. Luckily, human studies have also verified the benefits of probiotics for mood. In a double-blind, placebo-controlled, randomized parallel group study, a French team found that giving humans specific strains of lactobacillus and bifidobacterium for thirty days yielded beneficial psychological effects including lowered depression, less anger and hostility, and better problem solving, compared to the placebo group.

Yeast and Anxiety

Yeast (also known as candida) is fungus that can thrive in an unhealthy digestive tract. Known to be associated with blood sugar problems, poor immune system function, and fungal infections (like mouth thrush and toenail fungus), yeast can signify a microbiome that is out of balance.

While a healthy microbiome will contribute to good mood, an unhealthy one full of *Candida albicans,* and all the toxins associated with it, will contribute to mood disorder. Presence of this yeast will alter the gut's ability to absorb nutrients and push hypersensitivity reactions of toxic by-products, which translates to inflammation in the body. Inflammation will greatly contribute to anxiety and poor mental function.

Unhealthy microbiome → yeast buildup → toxic byproducts → hypersensitivity reactions → inflammation → mood problems (anxiety and depression)

There are many wonderful natural foods full of probiotics. Here is a list of probiotic foods to try.

- Natto (a traditional Japanese fermented food)
- Kim chi (Korean-style cabbage)
- Sauerkraut
- Yogurt
- Kefir
- Tempeh
- Fermented milk (like buttermilk)
- Miso
- Non-baked cheeses (like aged cheese)

Note: Homemade sauerkraut is better than the store-bought kind, because the store-bought stuff often undergoes pasteurization, a process that kills a lot of the good bacteria.

Crunchy Vegetables to Lower Anxiety

Ever notice how most people get pleasure from crunchy foods? Have you seen the commercial where the kid "can't eat just one"? There's a scientific reason for this: crunching makes people feel happier (when they are doing the crunching themselves—not so much when someone right next to you is the cruncher).

Furthermore, have you noticed how these crunchy, snacky foods can cause us to eat to excess? A person who normally doesn't eat a lot will end up eating the whole bag. This is called "hedonic hyperphagia"—a fancy term for when someone eats to excess because it feels good. To examine the effects of excessive pleasure eating, one astute German researcher used enhanced MRI technology on rats that were given either regular chow or crunchy snacks. He found that crunchy snacks activate more brain reward centers than the noncrunchy chow. Other research suggests that the crunching sound itself allows pleasure centers to release more endorphins. Since crunchy food is calming, it can help assuage anxiety.

Please note that I am not recommending that you pull out a bag of chips when you are anxious. Unfortunately, when we eat too many calories from junky-crunchy foods, we tend to feel even worse. So instead of unhealthy chips and cookies, try bringing in healthy crunchy foods: veggies like carrots, celery, and peppers. There are a number of healthy baked snacks, like flax meal crackers and high bran fiber crackers, that will also do the job. Nuts are great, too—but should be raw. The nice thing about these healthy snacks is that you will get the anxiety-lowering effect without overeating—it is really hard to overeat healthy foods.

Ideas for Healthy Crunch Foods:

- Baby carrots
- Dried crunchy vegetables: peas, carrots, peppers
- Celery with raw almond butter or natural peanut butter
- Raw nuts and seeds: almonds, walnuts, cashews, pumpkin seeds, sunflower seeds
- Baked flax crackers
- Bran and whole grain/fiber crackers—use gluten-free versions if sensitive
- Raw food crunch snacks: kale chips, veggie chips

Let's Go Nuts

Health-conscious people have eaten raw nuts for millennia. In addition to their crunchiness, nuts are chock full of healthy fatty acids and oils, as well as protein and minerals. Nuts have been studied for their ability to lower anxiety-producing inflammation in the body as well.

One study looked at levels of inflammatory markers in people who ate nuts regularly. These people had lower levels of C-reactive protein (CRP), a protein found in the blood when inflammation is high. This marker is strongly correlated with cardiovascular disease, and is likely a better predictor of heart and blood vessel problems than cholesterol. Other inflammation markers like the immune system component interleukin-6 (IL-6) and vascular adhesion factors (which make blood vessel walls too sticky) were also brought way down. CRP and IL-6 are typically quite high in people who have anxiety and depression. Most researchers believe that the benefits in nuts come from their healthy fatty acids and high magnesium levels, two anxiety-busting components.

Healthy raw nuts include almonds, Brazil nuts, chestnuts, and cashews. While toasted nuts are often eaten, I'd recommend going easy on them: heating the nut damages its oils, making it go rancid and rendering it unhealthful for the brain and body. If you prefer the taste of roasted nuts, try mixing two or three parts raw to one part roasted.

Unhealthy Food Choices for Mood

Just as healthy foods can help support a healthy nervous system and good mood, poor quality foods will work against your best health.

Before we talk about foods that are not so good for your mood, please note that we started the conversation about food with foods that are healthy. This was on purpose—I wanted to start by encouraging you to bring in healthy foods first. My patients have taught me this is the best approach. For most people, it is not effective to focus on what they cannot eat—they feel deprived and sometimes angry. You may feel the same. As a result, you may have a rebound reaction and end up eating even more of the "unhealthy" foods we would like to remove as a way to gain a sense of control over your anxiety. If you feel this way, just focus on healthy foods to add for now. As you add these great foods, you will feel better; later, you may want to consider reducing your intake of the foods that are not so good for your brain and body.

A Little Tasty Morsel about Taste

Research shows that the brain has a similar reaction to both something that is morally violating to an individual (like seeing a person kick a dog) and a taste that is unpleasant. So among the healthy foods, first pick the ones that you find pleasing and tasty—unpleasant tastes may exacerbate negative mood. I have found that as people feel better and eat more healthy foods, their palate expands and they are more willing to take risks with their diet.

Foods to Avoid

Some foods will work against you in your effort to beat anxiety for good. Just remember: no one has to be a saint all the time when it comes to food, but the more you work on this, the more your brain and body will respond.

High-Glycemic Foods

Sugary foods (juices, cakes, cookies, candy) and simple carbohydrate foods (white breads, bagels, pasta, white rice) are known as high-glycemic foods. They contain high levels of easily absorbed sugar, which triggers any disease to which you may be predisposed. This sugar can also contribute to diabetes, dementia, heart disease, and cancer.

High consumption of sugars and carbs can contribute to mood disorders not only by not providing important nutrients but also by depleting important minerals, like magnesium. Minerals are very important cofactors for the production of neurotransmitters and help minimize the effect of toxins that enter your body.

High-glycemic foods also trigger release of excess insulin. Insulin is the hormone whose job it is to move high levels of sugar out of the blood stream before the sugar crystals do too much damage to our tissues. Insulin also tends to drive inflammation, and as we have seen, brain inflammation contributes to mood problems. Higher insulin levels will also drop your blood sugar below normal levels and make you hungry. Hunger and hypoglycemia (low blood sugar) are primitive signals known to set off a stress response in the body. In people who are predisposed to anxiety, this is a very typical catalyst to a panic attack. More about blood sugar in a bit.

Unhealthy Fats

Which foods are most damaging to mood?

As we discussed, unhealthy fats—like hydrogenated oils, highly heated vegetable oil, fried foods, and non-grass-fed animal-based saturated fats are best avoided. Healthy fats will keep the membranes of your nervous system happy and fluid. Fluid membranes mean calm inflammatory pathways. Immune system cell membranes that lack fluidity also contribute to inflammation. When you eat more unhealthy fats, these cell membranes become rigid and do not allow nutrients to get in or toxins to get out. By eating unhealthy fats, you will push inflammation and prevent your body from cleansing itself—two things that will cause anxiety.

Food Additives

Food additives, like artificial colors, glutamate (MSG), and artificial sweeteners, have all been linked to mood problems. While there are supposedly strict governmental guidelines for food additives, their long-term safety has not been rigorously proven. The FDA has a very hands-off approach to food additives and does not do any testing itself—it lets the companies that make and sell these chemicals regulate their own safety. It is a bit like letting the fox tend the hen house.

As many of the parents of my younger patients can attest, color additives have been linked to conduct and mood disorder, as well as attention issues in kids. Recent animal studies showed that those taking both low- and high-dose tartrazine (known affectionately as FD and C Yellow No. 5) exhibited increased hyperactivity, with significant promotion of anxiety responses. Depression responses were also greatly heightened over animals not exposed to tartrazine. The authors concluded that the study "points to the hazardous impact of tartrazine on public health." Human studies from 1994 have also linked anxiety to these chemicals. Tartrazine is used in tons of foods that kids and adults eat every day: colored foods, candies, and even in medications. Stay away from these as much as you can.

Glutamate is an excitatory neurotransmitter the brain produces in small physiologic amounts as a by-product of everyday cell metabolism. Monosodium glutamate (MSG) is a special salt form of glutamate. While this compound does occur naturally in some foods in small amounts (including hydrolyzed vegetable protein, yeasts, soy extracts, protein isolate, cheese, and tomatoes), the additive MSG is used in high amounts primarily to enhance taste. I will admit, it does taste good—but I do not believe it's worth the cost to your mood.

Despite the fact that the FDA considers the additive MSG to be GRAS (generally recognized as safe), it is toxic to the brain and to your mood. In fact, excess glutamate is more cytotoxic to nerve cells than cyanide—studies show levels of glutamate in patients with mood disorder to be significantly higher than in healthy people. Have you ever had a reaction to Chinese food—maybe anxiety, low mood, headache, or a little stomach upset and nausea? It is not uncommon for Chinese food to contain MSG, and those who react to it might have a large store of glutamate already and/or are not able to detoxify it. While your brain uses a very sophisticated system to remove glutamate, and heavy metal burden will decrease the brain's ability to clear it out. People with anxiety (and humans in general) should avoid ingesting any of it.

Artificial sweeteners (such as saccharin, aspartame, sucralose, and acesulfame potassium) are also known to have toxic effects on the nervous system and may assault the neurotransmitters you need for your best mood. This is not new information: a 1984 paper in the *American Journal of Clinical Nutrition* revealed that aspartame may contribute to abnormal balance of the neurotransmitter serotonin. When the aspartame was removed, anxiety relief was reported in numerous cases; clear recurrence occurred when people started to eat it again. Just to be balanced, I will tell you that one large study in 2002 did find aspartame very "safe," with "no unresolved questions regarding its safety." However, you should know that this study, which was quoted all over the news media, was actually funded by the Nutrasweet Company—the people who make these toxins.

What About Coffee?

. . . coffee sets the blood in motion and stimulates the muscles;
it accelerates the digestive processes, chases away sleep,
and gives us the capacity to engage a little longer
in the exercise of our intellects.

—Honoré de Balzac

Conventional wisdom suggests that caffeine-containing drinks are considered a "no-no" when it comes to anxiety. There's good reason for this—but let's review the information about these caffeinated products in terms of mood issues and see what makes the most sense.

Let's start with coffee. Interestingly, when I first started getting anxiety and panic attacks in the early 1990s, sometimes the thought of driving four hours from Washington, DC where I was doing research at the National Institutes of Health, to get back to my parents' home in Staten Island, New York, was enough to cause panic for me. For whatever reason, I found that it really helped if I went to a coffee shop and picked up a large coffee for the ride home—I still felt anxious, but somehow happier and less panicky at the same time.

As the most well used psychoactive drug of all time, coffee is an interesting compound, with mixed reviews regarding its effect on health and mood. Regarding overall health, studies show some wonderful health effects for coffee. It can decrease a pre-diabetic's risk for diabetes, lower incidence of bile tract and liver cancer, and even help prevent heart attacks after a meal. In fact, a 2013 review of the larger epidemiologic studies show regular coffee consumption to reduce mortality, both for all-cause and cardiovascular deaths. In addition, coffee intake is associated with lower rates of heart failure, stroke, diabetes, and some cancers.

As far as anxiety is concerned, coffee can be both beneficial and harmful. For me, I found it helped with specific situational panic attacks, but could heighten my generalized anxiety if I drank too much. How will it affect you? As with many questions in holistic medicine, the answer is "it depends." If you are reading this and already know you are very caffeine-sensitive, let's honor that—you can skip to the next section.

The positive mood effects of coffee lie in caffeine's ability to increase the senses of euphoria and energy, which it did for me. Caffeine helps the brain release dopamine into the prefrontal cortex, an area important for mood regulation. In a ten-year cohort study of more than 50,000 older women, investigators found that compared to those who drank one cup or less of caffeinated coffee per week, those who drank two to three cups per day had a 15 percent decreased risk for depression, and those who drank four cups or more had a 20 percent decreased risk. I believe it may help situational anxiety and panic attacks because it raises levels of dopamine.

Dopamine is typically low in people with depression and social anxiety. Social anxiety is a type of situational anxiety. If you experience either of these, try drinking coffee daily (or just before the situation of stress or panic). Of course, if you try coffee and find that it makes you feel worse, or you stop sleeping, then it is not the beverage for you.

Please note: there is a threshold to coffee's benefit, even in people with severe depression and low dopamine. Another study from Finland found that although the risk for suicide decreased progressively for those consuming up to seven cups of coffee per day, the risk started increasing when consumption went over eight cups a day. Also noteworthy is that decaffeinated coffee, caffeinated tea, and chocolate did *not* have positive effects. And even when used for social anxiety and depression, long-term coffee use will still contribute to "burnout" in people who are already depleted and deficient. Caffeine is a mood-boosting substance, but too much, even for people who can tolerate it, will turn things very bad moodwise.

There are other negative health effects: caffeine at long-term high doses can encourage mineral loss, such as magnesium, which is an important cofactor for brain neurotransmitters. Coffee may also contribute to fluctuations in blood sugar, which can raise anxiety levels. As you may already know, caffeine-sensitive individuals may experience more insomnia. As we learned earlier, poor sleep will promote both anxiety and depression in predisposed individuals. Again, whether coffee is best for you really depends on your particular situation. You may not want to start drinking coffee until you have worked on your sleep, diet, and lifestyle.

What about Green Tea?
Originally used by the Chinese monks over 4,700 years ago, green tea was known to help these religious men attain a state of "relaxed wakefulness" while meditating. While the tea's caffeine content is likely responsible for keeping them from falling asleep while meditating, there are two other components that may account for its

Healthful Foods to Increase

+ Mediterranean diet foods
+ Fish
+ Raw nuts and seeds
+ Probiotic foods
+ Crunchy vegetables

Foods to Avoid

+ High-glycemic foods (sugary foods and simple carbohydrates)
+ Unhealthy saturated fats
+ Food additives: MSG, dyes, FDA colors, artificial sugars

Coffee: Best for depressive moods, avoid with general anxiety and insomnia. Possibly beneficial for social anxiety and panic.

Green tea: Okay for low mood and depression; might be okay for anxiety patients who are not caffeine-sensitive.

relaxation effect. Animal studies on the polyphenol epigallocatechin gallate (EGCG), which is present in green tea, suggest that it relieves anxiety by turning on the GABA receptors in the brain—these are the same receptors that anxiety-relieving drugs like Xanax target. Also, green tea has theanine, a naturally contained amino acid that has anxiety-improving and blood pressure-lowering effects.

Generally, coffee is beneficial for you if you are susceptible to low mood, low motivation, and depression. But if you have generalized anxiety disorder, sleeping problems, or general caffeine sensitivity, it will probably make things worse. Coffee may be useful for treating social phobia and even panic attacks in some people. The only way to know if it is right for you is to try it—in a safe setting, of course. Green tea can be helpful for both anxiety and depression, but, like coffee, I would start slowly and see how you feel. Do not overdo it, and if there is any worsening of anxiety or sleep issues, stop right away.

Inflammation, Leaky Gut, and Mood

The majority of the body's immune system is housed in the digestive tract (mucosa-associated lymphoid tissue [MALT] and gut-associated lymphoid tissue [GALT]). Stress combined with poor digestion often leads to an activation of the inflammatory components of the immune system, which leads to inflammation. Also, ingestion of charred, fried, and overly cooked foods creates molecules called advanced glycation end products (AGEs). These AGEs will also increase inflammation. As we have seen, inflammation will travel to the brain and contribute to anxiety; this is the reason why psychiatric problems are much more prevalent in patients with intestinal inflammatory conditions. Junk food and processed foods will also disturb healthy digestion.

Significantly greater amounts of inflammation are present in people with anxiety. Inflammation markers in your immune system, such as C-reactive protein (CRP), interleukin (IL-6), and tumor-necrosis factor (TNF), correlate to anxiety, brain changes, and other body tissues. Inflammation contains the word "flame"—and too much inflammation, like a fire out of control, burns and destroys what's in its path. In the brain, it causes havoc. While anxiety seems to be a common manifestation of this inflammatory firefight in the body, depending on another person's particular predisposition and individual genetics, this process will contribute to practically any health issue to which a person might be predisposed.

With your firefight in the brain, you might have anxiety, but your friend's firefight might end up in the joints, and he will get rheumatoid arthritis. In the blood vessels, inflammation can cause coronary artery disease, which is the leading cause of heart attacks. If the firefight goes to the skin, then inflammation there manifests as eczema, psoriasis, and acne. Kidney and lung inflammation will show up as lupus and other organ problems, while various tissue inflammations are known propagators of cancer. Nondescript inflammation in the muscles will reveal itself as fibromyalgia and chronic fatigue. Inflammation that stays in the digestive tract will cause inflammatory bowel disease (like Crohn's disease or ulcerative colitis). These will both contribute to more digestive issues and inflammation.

As you may be starting to figure out, almost every disease has an inflammatory component. And it is likely that every inflammation has a digestive and stress component. This is why naturopathic physicians believe food and digestion is vitally important to consider when working on virtually any health problem.

In the 1990s, I was part of a research team in Bethesda, Maryland, at the National Institutes of Health. Part of our work was to use animal studies to figure out which immune components might be turned on in the brain when the body was stressed out and inflamed. Up until then, the brain's immune system was not well documented. In fact, many medical professionals considered the brain to be a privileged and protected organ that didn't have any immune cells at all. In our research, we gave these cute little white rats regular doses of a bacterial coat compound called lipopolysaccharide (LPS) as a way to ramp up inflammation. The rat immune system "sees" this bacterial coat and prompts a strong inflammatory response, and the inflamed animals showed "sickness behavior," which included fatigue, anxiety, and hyperactivity. After a while, the rats started to show low mood, low motivation, and other symptoms and signs that clearly correlate with anxiety and depression. This is exactly what happens to humans when there are high levels of inflammation. To me, this was important research, for it showed us that inflammation in the body causes major mood problems—the same problems that almost 25 percent of Americans face every day.

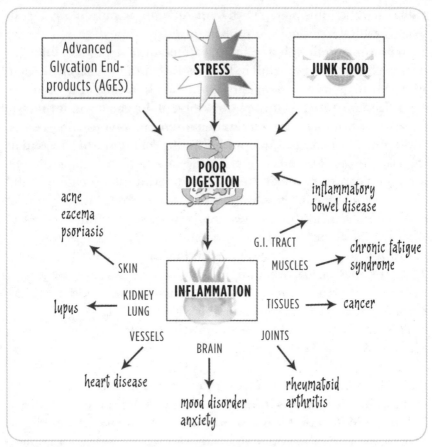

Figure 5.1: Inflammation's contribution to health problems

What Is Intestinal Permeability and Leaky Gut, Exactly?

For the past few decades, holistic practitioners like myself have referred to a concept called "leaky gut" as being a fundamental connection between poor digestion and inflammation-derived disease. While the rats I mentioned above might experience inflammation from a dose of bacteria, in humans, certain foods can spark immune-related responses in the digestive tract. This response will cause inflammatory reactions throughout the rest of the body.

Stress will also increase the likelihood of immune responses by inhibiting proper digestive enzyme production. When you are not making enough digestive enzymes, your food doesn't break down; when your food doesn't break down, larger than normal particles of food reach the intestines. These particles look weird to the immune system, and in an attempt to protect the body from absorbing them, the immune system will get all irritable and inflamed.

If you and a friend spent ten seconds lobbing grenades at each other in an apartment building, you might bust a few holes in the walls, yes? Your neighbors would call the police, you would be arrested, and maybe a few days later the super would patch things up. Right? Now, let's say you and a friend spend all day, every day lobbing grenades. What would happen to the walls of the apartment? You would blow holes in them, and the super would not have enough time to fix it. This is what happens in your intestines when you eat problem foods: your immune system is constantly lobbing chemical bombs around and your body doesn't have time to clean up the mess.

Long-term inflammation in your digestive tract over a period of time will significantly compromise both the structure and repair mechanisms of the digestive tract. Under this inflammatory fire, tight junctions known to hold digestive tract cells together begin to deteriorate. When these structures break down, material in the space of the gastrointestinal tract has greater access to the bloodstream. This is known as "gut permeability" or simply "leaky gut." Other items can trigger this breakdown, too, like antibiotics, food preservatives, and toxins. Even exercise causes a temporary leaky gut that repairs itself (except in cases where the body is overextended). Besides the tight junctions becoming shredded, the fingerlike projections called villi on cell surfaces are also damaged, leading to poor nutrient absorption.

Particles that escape from the digestive tract will get into the bloodstream, travel to the rest of the body and cause whole-body inflammatory effects, which in turn will contribute to eventual disease. As we discussed in the last section, if someone has a predisposition to disease, leaky gut and its accompanying inflammation will increase the likelihood that this disease will become a problem. For you, this means more anxiety.

While leaky gut is fairly well recognized in natural medicine and CAM circles, conventional biomedicine has spurned the concept, calling it the unproven work of pseudoscientists. Even though this attitude is very common, it seems to fly in the face of solid medical research.

Indeed, the research suggests that leaky gut syndrome is quite real and is a strong contributor to disease—including mood disorder. One

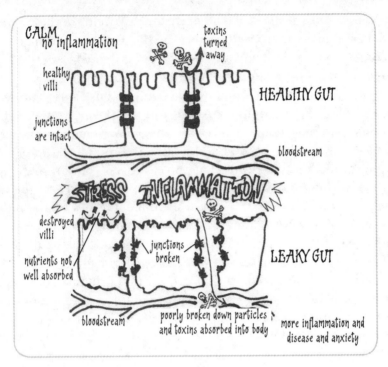

Figure 5.2: Leaky gut

2008 study looked at the serum concentrations of antibodies immunoglobulin M and G, or IgM and IgG, in chronic fatigue patients. The presence of these antibodies indicates that bacteria leaked from the digestive tract into the blood. These antibodies pretty much serve as markers of a leaky gut—if the gut wasn't leaking, the bacteria would not be in the blood, causing the antibodies to form. Forty-one of these chronic fatigue patients were given a leaky gut diet and were prescribed natural anti-inflammatory and antioxidative supplements such as glutamine, n-acetyl cysteine (NAC), and zinc. After an average of ten to fourteen months, twenty-four patients showed a significant clinical improvement or remission and normalization of the immune responses. Their mood improved, too. This study joins reams of other studies in cardiovascular journals, liver journals, kidney journals, and of course digestive tract publications, all of which discuss leaky gut in association with chronic disease. There is a test to see if you have leaky gut. It is called the lactulose-mannitol test, and can be ordered through your naturopathic doctor. I find it's very valuable to help my patients identify an important contributor to anxiety and many other health problems.

Gluten "Allergy" versus Gluten "Sensitivity"

We know that our inability to break down unhealthy food can cause inflammation. But I have seen many patients who are eating healthy diets, yet they are having digestive and anxiety problems. How can this be? Following the axiom "one man's food may be another man's poison," this section will explore why some people have trouble with traditionally healthy foods.

"Food allergy" refers to an overt immune system response that results in creation of immune antibodies. This is the kind of response that can lead to throat closing or tremendous swelling (called anaphylaxis). While any food can trip this off in a predisposed individual, the most common food allergies are shellfish, nuts, fish, milk, peanuts, and eggs. Celiac disease is also an allergy situation where there is an autoimmune response to gluten (a protein present in wheat, rye, and barley).

"Food sensitivity" or "food intolerance" is a subtler response that occurs in the digestive tract, often occurring when foods are not well digested, and spurs unwanted inflammatory reactions.

The nervous system is vulnerable to the ravages of food reaction. Neurological manifestations in patients with established celiac disease have been reported since 1966. However, it was not until thirty years later that gluten sensitivity was shown to manifest not so much in the digestive system, but instead solely in the nervous system, causing problems such as unexplained neuropathies (strange sensations in feet, hands, and other body parts) and ataxia (uncoordinated muscle movements). We now know that these under-the-radar reactions can also cause mood problems.

Celiac disease is an antibody-mediated disease affecting 1 percent of the population. It is generally characterized by gastrointestinal complaints, and if it goes on long enough, weight loss. Gluten sensitivities, however, cause much subtler reactions, often without overt gastrointestinal problems or weight loss, and will likely manifest as nervous system problems and psychiatric symptoms—maybe even anxiety.

The subtle gluten sensitivities I am talking about occur a whopping six times (that's 600 percent) more often than actual celiac disease, and, unlike celiac, there are no antibody tests to identify these sensitivities. When I suspect patients have these sensitivities and I recommend they stop eating gluten foods, they often see marked improvement in mood and digestive tract symptoms. In 2013, doctors in Italy published a paper entitled "Non-Celiac Gluten Sensitivity: The New Frontier of Gluten Related Disorders." In it, they discuss exactly how gluten and other components of wheat can cause low-grade inflammatory issues in the digestive tract, like irritable bowel syndrome, and contribute to a number of diseases, including mood disorders.

Besides gluten, there may be other foods—even healthy foods—that can also contribute to sensitivity reactions. In my clinic, I have found two approaches can help identify subtle food sensitivities. One is working with Dr. Peter D'Adamo's blood type diet. Eating foods appropriate for your blood type can help limit your sensitivity responses. The blood type diet takes into account the little proteins that sit on the top of your immune cells (*glycoproteins*) and how they are affected by food proteins (*lectins*). The basic approach suggests that everyone should eat mostly whole foods and healthful vegetables. But depending on your blood type, you will want to focus on eating certain foods that are extra healthy, and avoid foods that drive inflammation. For example, people who have type A blood should eat plenty of salmon, pineapple, pumpkin seeds, and berries, while avoiding red meat, dairy products, and tomatoes. People who are type O do very well with cod, grass-fed beef, and kale, and should try to minimize dairy products and gluten. Blood type B people do well with most dairy, lamb, and flounder, but need to avoid chicken and shellfish. Blood type AB patients do well with broccoli, grapefruits, yogurt, and lamb, but may need to stay away from beef and certain beans. While no single dietary approach is 100 percent accurate for everyone, the blood type diet has worked well for my patients. See appendix II for resources to get started with the blood type diet.

A second approach is the elimination challenge diet. This involves removing foods that are typically the most reactive (like dairy, soy, corn, wheat/gluten, eggs, peanuts, citrus, alcohol, and caffeine) for four to six weeks. Over this time, your anxiety and physical symptoms may resolve or decrease significantly. Once this happens, you add back one food every four days and look for a reaction (like anxiety, panic, headache, itchiness, skin reaction, heart racing . . .). Any food that elicits this reaction may be an inflammatory food for you. Visit my website, *www.drpeterbongiorno.com/eliminationdiet,* where I will walk you through an elimination challenge program.

If your symptoms do not resolve or if you are just reactive to absolutely everything, then you may need to first follow the below steps to healing an inflamed gut, and then retry the elimination diet protocol.

How to Heal Your Inflamed Gut

As illustrated in figure 5.1, the body tells us it's on fire in various ways: skin conditions like rashes, eczema, psoriasis, rosacea; or internal conditions such as cancer, autoimmune conditions, cardiovascular disease, mental illness, or inflammatory bowel disease. Blood tests that reveal high levels of ESR, CRP, homocysteine, and/or autoimmune markers can point to inflammation. You can use these physical tests and blood markers help to decide if you are inflamed and, if so, how much.

Here is your program to de-inflame and get your brain calm.

Meditation, Relaxation, Mind-Body Work
Do this work to help increase parasympathetic response and support circulation to the digestive tract. The next chapter will talk about this work.

Sleep Work
Aim for eight hours of sleep, getting to bed by 11:00 p.m. at the latest to help balance immune function. Please refer to chapter 3 for more help with sleep.

Exercise
Work out at least three times a week for a half hour to burn stress hormones and calm the nervous system. You'll build muscle to support insulin sensitivity, thus lowering the inflammation-producing insulin hormone. See chapter 4 for more information about exercise.

Food Work
Focus on the Mediterranean diet: fish, green vegetables, raw nuts and seeds, and plenty of fiber. Cut down on foods with chemicals,

preservatives, and dyes. Limit red meats and avoid dairy, gluten, and foods cooked at high temperatures. Consider following the blood type diet or try the elimination diet program for four weeks.

Supplements

To help lower inflammation and heal a leaky gut:

Probiotics are beneficial to heal the mucosal membrane. Dosages will vary with preparation. We use Restoraflora in our clinic.

Zinc. Studies of patients with Crohn's disease (a serious inflammatory disease of the intestine) have shown that zinc supplementation can resolve permeability alterations and help prevent relapse in patients who are in remission. Typical dose is 15 mg twice a day of zinc carnosine.

Curcumin. This wonder herb helps decrease inflammation and oxidative stress in the gut. Dosage will depend on preparation and is best in between meals. More about curcumin in chapter 7.

Glutamine is a preferred fuel for digestive tract cells and helps with repair of the intestines. Standard dosage is one teaspoon twice a day in liquid, away from meals.

Roberts Formula is an old naturopathic formula (AKA Bastyr formula) with anecdotal efficacy for healing the digestive tract. This is my go-to formula to help heal the gut. Unfortunately, no formal research has been done on this herbal combination. While there are variations, the standard formula usually includes althea, echinacea, ulmus, geranium, phytolacca, hydrastis, and cabbage powder. Cabbage is high in glutamine. Some versions also include niacinamide and pancreatic enzymes. Typical dosage is two capsules three times a day in between meals.

Small Intestinal Bacterial Overgrowth

As we have learned, poor digestion leads to anxiety. Another intestinal issue that may contribute to anxiety is small intestinal bacterial overgrowth (SIBO). This is a condition where bad bacteria in the small intestine can grow to excess; it can even move up into the stomach. SIBO can also contribute to irritable bowel syndrome as well as lactose and fructose intolerances. For my patients with symptoms of anxiety along with digestive distress such as belching, gas, and flatulence, I recommend a SIBO test. This simple, non-invasive test involves blowing into a tube a couple of times over a few hours after eating a very simple diet for twenty-four hours. By looking at the buildup of certain gases that will show up in your breath, we can learn if SIBO is an issue for you. In most cases, once the bacteria is treated and cleaned out, the anxiety cleans out with it. Treatment includes using herbal medicines like oregano, garlic, and berberine. Patients are also encouraged to follow the FODMAP (fermentable oligo-di-monosaccharides and polyols) diet, and in some cases, to take a type of antibiotic called Rifaximin. Following treatment with herbs and/or an antibiotic also entails the use of probiotics. The lab I use to check for SIBO is Commonwealth Labs, at *www.hydrogenbreathtesting.com.*

Blood Sugar

I have strange blood sugar levels. I get very odd if I don't eat. I either want to hit someone, cry, or fall asleep.
—Alison Goldfrapp

Blood sugar regulation is key to managing and beating anxiety of all types. Way back in 1938, Dr. John Quinlan, a San Francisco doctor, first published his research showing the relationship between low blood sugar and anxiety. When your blood sugar is out of whack, your body's stress system turns up. It's as simple as that, and it makes a lot of sense.

When there are dips in blood sugar, the primitive brain thinks, "hey, we are going to starve here," and starts sending a distress signal to the body to stop thinking or doing anything else and just worry about the next meal. While our animal brains have "evolved" to the point where hunger doesn't make us drop on all fours and search for food anymore, this response still makes us stressed out, and often we don't even realize it. Studies of subjects who have wild fluctuations in blood sugar show that these patients develop brain and cognitive difficulties, and experience lots of sadness and anxiety—anxiety that is avoidable.

Have you ever met (or lived with) anyone who gets "hangry" (that's hungry plus angry) when she goes too long without eating? That is a form of the blood sugar stress response. I have known my wife for almost twenty years now. When we first met, it was clear to me that when she was hungry, her mood changed—sometimes dramatically. It was not fun. As soon as she ate, she returned to her sweet self (and usually, but not always, an apology followed). Now she knows better than to let herself get hangry, so she carries a little snack with her for emergencies.

We will discuss blood tests that look closely at blood sugar in appendix I. These tests may give you insight into how your blood sugar functions. Either way, if you notice that you get more anxious when you don't eat, I highly recommend following the recommendations below. Even if you do not think blood sugar variations affect you, try these suggestions anyway. I have seen many cases of anxious patients who eat three good meals a day. When I place them on a five to six small meal schedule, their anxiety lets up considerably.

Also, if you know your blood sugar is off, you may want to keep a blood sugar diary to illustrate the relationship between your anxiety symptoms and your blood sugar levels. I find this most valuable—some of my patients seem to have more issues early in the day, while others have trouble right before meals or in the evening. Knowing when your challenges occur will help you better understand when and how much to eat to control the anxiety response.

If your blood sugar is off, try the following steps:

1. Cut out all simple carbohydrate foods and sugary foods. This includes white breads, bagels, pasta (as a Sicilian, I can tell you that's not an easy one), cookies, cakes, sodas, and juices. Even diet sodas are known to mess up metabolism and blood sugar, so those need to go, too. These foods will bring your sugar up fast, which will make your pancreas increase insulin, which will drop your sugar even more, putting you on the hyperglycemia/hypoglycemia yo-yo.

2. Start eating breakfast. At the risk of sounding like your mother, breakfast really is the most important meal of the day. Research shows that when you eat a good breakfast with plenty of protein, your insulin responses are much more balanced over the course of the day. No more yo-yo. See appendix IV for a list of some of the best breakfast food choices.

3. Eat every three hours. Aim for small, frequent meals that have protein, healthy fat, and healthy carbs.

4. Take some blood sugar supportive supplements. Chromium is a mineral that helps balance blood sugar. Try 200 mcg (mcg stands for micrograms—a microgram is one thousandth of a milligram) three times a day with meals. Cinnamon can help you balance sugars, too. Take one teaspoon in the morning, in tea or oatmeal. We will talk more about these in chapter 7.

put anxiety behind you

5. Adequate sleep, exercise, and stress management are also important to help your body balance blood sugar.

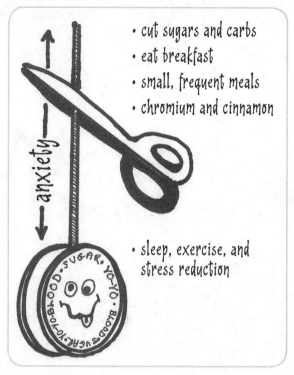

• cut sugars and carbs
• eat breakfast
• small, frequent meals
• chromium and cinnamon

• sleep, exercise, and stress reduction

Figure 5.3: Stop blood sugar yo-yo

Checklist for Digestive Health

❏ Fix constipation. Water, fiber, stress reduction, natural laxatives if needed

❏ Create healthier digestion. Breathing, bitters, chew well, healthy foods, relaxation work

❏ Good food choices. Mediterranean diet, plenty of protein, probiotic foods, avoid unhealthy foods

❏ Fix leaky gut. Meditation, sleep, exercise, healthy foods and elimination diet, supplementation

❏ Control blood sugar fluctuations. Avoid simple carbs, eat breakfast, eat regularly (every three hours), consume chromium and cinnamon, get enough sleep, exercise, and stress reduction work

6

mind-body therapy

Nothing can bring you peace but yourself.
—Ralph Waldo Emerson

Case: Med Student Shana

Shana was a young medical student recently admitted to a top medical school in New York City. Even though she was brilliant, she had had a tough time getting into med school because of her general anxiety and especially her nervousness around test-taking. Now she was at the school of her dreams, but within the first few months, she was in danger of failing out due to her test-taking anxiety.

When I met her, I was amazed at her spark, intelligence, and quick thinking. She talked a mile a minute, almost to the point where I couldn't quite understand the words. I asked her if she was especially nervous, and she said, "Nope, I'm okay. Why do you ask?"

We talked about a lot of things. I learned that she ate a fair amount of sugar and carb-y foods but very little protein, and she exercised a lot. She was "on" from the moment she got up

until the moment she collapsed into bed. I developed a plan for her to eat a good breakfast with lots of protein, lower her exercise a tad, and start taking the amino acid GABA, which has a calming effect. I had her start regular walks in the park, too. I also recommended she start meditating. When I mentioned meditation, her first reaction was "I hate that stuff."

When patients tell me they hate meditating, I know they need it the most. I explain how meditation brings you into a moment and allows the body's physiology to relax (after all, there is no bear running after it). When we met, Shana was in constant fight-or-flight mode, so she was always running from that fictitious bear.

We started with thirty seconds of meditation together in the office that day. It was hard for Shana at first, but she got it. We had to work on some of the thoughts that came up for her— themes that revolved around failure. We moved the meditation to one minute twice a day at home. Now, Shana is in her fourth year of medical school, and leads meditation classes for first- year students! Shana's generalized anxiety has calmed considerably, and she no longer stresses about tests.

In chapter 2, we talked about the cerebral cortex, the outer area of the brain. This is where we do our high-level thinking, and it is the part of the brain that makes us (supposedly) smarter than other animals. The cerebral cortex also causes us to overthink, and sends signals to our hypothalamus and amygdala (the fear center of the brain) to cause anxious feelings. As we have seen, this system is designed to help us recognize and escape danger. That is a good thing—when we are in danger. Unfortunately, those of us with anxiety tend to use this system a little too creatively and way too often. As a result, we can end up feeling like we are in danger when we really are not.

Luckily, there are wonderful, calming ways to help reset this system—to let your body know it is no longer in danger. While there are more methods to relieve stress than I can count, I will focus on the ones I have relied on personally and that I see work most often for my anxious patients. Alongside the writing and negative thought work you learned in chapter 2, these will be invaluable to your anxiety-free journey.

Sunlight

In this modern age, we tend to run from the sun due to what I believe to be understandable but overblown concerns about skin cancer. Since the time of the Greeks, heliotherapy (sun therapy) has been a valuable way to heal the body and balance the mind. Hippocrates, the father of medicine, recognized that people with mood challenges need plenty of sunlight.

Three ways healthful exposure to sunlight can calm and balance mood are by maintaining healthy levels of serotonin, balancing your circadian rhythm, and building up your vitamin D stores. John Denver sang "Sunshine, on my shoulder, makes me happy." While I am not sure he ran a full human research trial on this, he did seem to have a clear understanding of sunlight's benefit on mood.

When the eye is exposed to sunlight, the hypothalamus is activated. The hypothalamus houses your bodily clock and is also the meeting point for your nervous system, immune system, and hormonal system. Throughout your day, your rhythmic balance is highly dependent on the timing and length of sunlight exposure. So, getting the right amount of both light and darkness is key to creating circadian rhythms consistent with a healthy body and good mood. Traditional Chinese Medicine (TCM) is based on the notion of balancing the yin and yang—yin represents darkness and nighttime, while yang represents light and daytime. In TCM, you cannot have true health without balance between yin and yang. In the sleep section, we touched on the essential role darkness plays for our circadian health. Now we are going to discuss the benefits of light.

The Light Exposure and Serotonin Connection

Serotonin is a feel-good neurotransmitter that calms and improves mood at the same time. Levels of serotonin increase when there is more light around. This is probably why people are generally happier in the summertime. Indeed, one 2002 study that looked at the blood of 101 men showed that serotonin levels are at their lowest in the winter. Even more, the rate of serotonin production in the brain and body depends on how long a person was exposed to light, as well how strong the light was (the strength of the light is known as intensity). This is why sunlight exposure in the summer is generally more effective than in the winter. Other studies have also shown how serotonin transporters (little proteins that bind up and inactivate serotonin) are more plentiful in the brain during dark periods. Darkness sends a signal to our bodies to keep things "low." If you are predisposed to anxiety and your serotonin is generally low, then you're extremely likely to suffer from anxiety and panic.

Sunlight and Circadian Rhythm

Modern life has given us infinite ways to keep the sun away from our skin. During the day, most of us stay indoors to work. We are clothed from top to bottom. Even when we are outside traveling, we stay in vehicles that block the sun. Our environment is becoming one big sun blocker—even air pollution blocks what used to be healthful sun exposure. Even more, modern medicine has all but scared us into blocking the last bit of sunlight we might accidentally receive by telling us to use sunblock.

Your body needs exposure to light—especially in the morning hours. But let's face it: how often do you get outdoors in the morning? Probably not while you're rushing to work or school. I know that even when I go for a run outside in the morning, unless it's summer, I run in the dark anyway! It's hard for a fellow to catch a sun break. As we have discussed, this minimal sun exposure is detrimental to our circadian rhythm, which needs high levels of morning cortisol (an adrenal stress hormone). The body generally decreases its cortisol production as the day goes on, with the lowest levels in the evening (see appendix I). When the sun goes down and cortisol is low, melatonin is properly secreted into the body. This sends a gentle but firm signal to the nervous system to calm down, unwind, relax—it is time to sleep.

When you do not get enough sun, your circadian rhythm gets out of whack, with cortisol levels fluctuating inappropriately throughout the day (more about this in appendix I). When these stress hormones pop up and down at the wrong time, the body knows that the clock in the hypothalamus and the whole stress system is off kilter. You will be more likely to experience anxiety and mood problems.

Mood disorder has been clearly associated with delayed release of melatonin, which will happen when cortisol is too high at night, and/or when you go to bed too late. If you are a "morning type," good for you—your hours support a healthy circadian rhythm. Morning people find they want to fall asleep between nine and ten at night and wake up by five or six. So-called "morning people" are more likely to get out in the early hours to enjoy morning bright light exposure, decreased morning melatonin secretion, more healthful circadian rhythms, and less anxiety.

Sunlight and Vitamin D

Sunlight is a major source of vitamin D, which is crucial for many of your body processes. Low vitamin D levels correlate with increases in risk of death from cancer, heart disease, and lung problems. Doctors advise their patients to stay out of the sun to reduce skin cancer deaths, but fear of the sun is likely causing more deaths from all other diseases—and it's contributing to mood problems.

Natural sunlight is actually made up of three light rays: visible light, ultraviolet light (UV light), and infrared radiation (IR). A component of UV light, UVB light, is responsible for catalyzing the conversion process that makes vitamin D in your skin by transforming a chemical called cutaneous 7-dehydrocholesterol into vitamin D3.

While UVB's ability to make vitamin D may be important, sunlight's infrared wavelengths also play an important role in mood. Research shows that when animals are exposed to infrared light and subjected to stressful tests, they are less likely to feel overcome with anxiety. In my office, I often combine acupuncture treatments with the use of an infrared device called a Teding Diancibo Pu lamp (commonly referred to as a TDP lamp). I have patients expose body parts such as the abdomen or lower back to this lamp, which emits heat and far-infrared light. Patients tell me that the TDP treatment helps them feel calm, secure, and nourished—and it warms them during their acupuncture session.

The take-home message from this section on sunlight? Get out in the sun when you can. Of course, don't overdo it and get a sunburn—it is true that too much sunlight will increase your risk of skin cancer. A good rule of thumb is to get out into the sun and expose your skin just until it starts to pink up a little bit. For more information about vitamin D testing and supplementing, see the vitamin D section in appendix I.

Early Morning Light: Light Box

While it's ideal to get your sunlight exposure from the sun itself, not everyone can do so safely. If you have very fair skin or a personal or family history of skin cancer, check with your doctor. You may need to opt for vitamin D supplementation or a phototherapy light box.

Light box therapy is known to be helpful for seasonal affective disorder (known affectionately as SAD). But it's also valuable for my patients with low cortisol levels in the morning and high levels at night (measure your levels with the adrenal saliva profile). The light box will help raise morning cortisol and reset this stress hormone to lower levels at night. Balanced cortisol will lower anxiety response, balance sugar control, and even help with lowering food cravings and the tendency to overeat.

If you decide to try the light box, look for a 10,000 lux full-spectrum white light. Sit in front of the light for at least thirty minutes every morning (see appendix II for light box info). My patients like to read, journal, or have a cup of tea in the morning while they use the light box.

Nature Medicine

A premise of naturopathic medicine is the principle that "nature heals." As a practitioner, this principle challenges me to bring to each patient the most natural methods to achieve healing and balance in the body. One powerful way to do this is to ask each patient to spend time in nature—and I am asking you to do the same thing right now.

Is nature therapy really helpful? Millions of people live in cities and they seem okay, right? In Traditional Chinese Medicine, healing occurs when you rebalance your body's energy with the energy of the environment around you. The idea is that nature knows how to stay in balance, and your body is a reflection of nature—so if your body goes out of whack, nature can help bring it back. In fact, the concept of feng shui suggests that if the energy in your home is out of balance, it will negatively affect your health. I know that when the room I'm in is neat, I feel better.

If it is true that our health is affected by the nature around us, we must ask ourselves: what happens when the environment is not healthy, and what does it do to the body? There are entire books on the subject of environmental medicine (the study of how toxins in the environment affect human health). The fact that our health is closely linked to our environment is why so many healthcare providers nowadays are passionate about saving the trees. They know that if we do not keep nature up and running, our health doesn't stand a chance.

One fascinating study compared the recoveries of gall bladder surgery patients. Members of one group had a bedside window view of trees; the other group's members looked out on a brick wall. The results showed that those with the nature view had shorter hospital stays and suffered fewer minor post-surgical problems, such as persistent headache or nausea. Furthermore, members of the nature group were more likely to be in good spirits, as reported by the hospital staff. The brick wall group did a lot more complaining—the staff gave evaluations that said things like "the patient is upset" and "patient needs much encouragement." Even more impressive: the patients with the tree view needed far fewer doses of strong narcotic pain medicines.

The Japanese have a very strong reverence and appreciation for nature. Their practice of spending time in nature is called forest bathing (or *shinrin-yoku*). This forest immersion is known for its health benefits, notably for mental health and the immune system. This treatment is simple—patients visit a forest and breathe in the air, which has molecules given off by the trees.

A study conducted by the Nippon Medical School in 2009 looked at twelve healthy men, ages thirty-seven through fifty-five. These men took a three-day, two-night trip through nature. During the trip, the subjects gave blood and urine samples at various intervals. On the first day, subjects walked through a forest field for two hours in the afternoon. On the second day, they walked through two different forest fields for two hours in the morning and afternoon. Blood samples from the second and third days showed that the immune cells known as "natural killer cells" and other anticancer factors were greatly increased. Moreover, the natural killer cell levels stayed elevated for a whole thirty days after the trip—pretty potent medicine. In addition, and likely more important for you, this study found that levels of the stress hormone adrenaline, which the body releases in response to anxiety, dropped down after forest bathing trips. I know that when I take a walk or run through the forest, I generally feel calm for the rest of the day.

Trees and plants give out various chemicals that are likely responsible for these positive effects on the body. Plants emit chemical aromas called phytoncides, which are organic antimicrobial molecules that may be responsible for both the calming and immune supportive effects of the forest.

Other research with seniors has shown how spending time in the forest will lower cortisol, blood pressure, heart rate, and inflammation in the body. At the same time, forest exposure kicks up your parasympathetic activity, which is the relaxation "rest and digest" response in the body—this is the response that is so needed to bring balance when you tend to be anxious.

A Multimodal Mood Study

I did my medical training at Bastyr University in Seattle. I am honored to say that Bastyr is considered to be on the top of the pile when it comes to naturopathic medicine and holistic education. Nearby University of Washington is a very prestigious conventional medical school, considered one of the best primary care medical programs in the country—but it's not a holistic school. Nevertheless, while I was in school in 2001, University of Washington researchers published what might be my favorite study of all time. It looked at 112 women with mild or moderate depression. Researchers asked the women to walk outside during daylight hours for twenty minutes five days a week. Subjects also took a multiple vitamin (which included vitamin B1 50 mg, some vitamin B2 and vitamin B6, folic acid 400 mcg, vitamin D 400 IU, and 200 mcg of selenium). A control group did not do any walking and received a placebo vitamin. The study found that 85 percent of the walking group felt less depression and anxiety, with greater self-esteem and well-being. That result is better than any antidepressant medication result to date.

This study was special because it paved the way for a new method of examining health and medicine. It changed a number of parameters at the same time, using lifestyle, nature, and vitamins together. Conventional research tends to look at one intervention (usually a drug) that is designed to stop a body process. For example, a person has reflux, he takes "the little purple pill," then the reflux is gone. Well, the reflux is gone because that little pill stops all acid production. That's good to get rid of acid reflux, but not good if you want your body to fix the problem and absorb nutrients. A naturopathic treatment would involve changing diet, working on stress, starting to exercise, and using supplements that help balance the stomach and its function, not suppress it. See the difference? This multiperspective, body-supportive approach needs to become the dominant way of doing research, for the better health of everyone. Another pioneer, Dr. Dean Ornish, has published studies in the *Journal of the American Medical Association* that involve a number of healthy changes, including aerobic exercise, stress management, smoking cessation, and group psychosocial support. After one year, Ornish showed that patients with heart problems had reversal of the atherosclerosis when they followed this multifactorial approach, whereas those patients following usual care only got worse! In five years, results were even better. Applying this health protocol to prostate cancer, Ornish found reversal of cancer genes turning on in men at both one and five years. These are truly amazing results—and unheard of in conventional care.

Ornish's work is the future of medicine. From my own experience over ten years, I can tell you that this perspective is also at the heart of what the best holistic medicine can offer patients with anxiety.

Your Indoor Environment

We talked about the benefits of being outside and how trees and plants communicate healthy things to your body. Well, bringing these green creatures inside, or even having pictures of them indoors, can also be beneficial. In fact, the images and things you keep around you in general will play a role in how you feel.

Because of this, I always recommend that my patients be careful about their indoor environment. Do this: whenever you have a say about what is around you, do your best to pick calming and positive images as much as possible. Studies show the benefit of having indoor houseplants in order to create a calming and healing environment.

Studies at Texas A&M in the 1980s looked at 160 heart recovery patients. Some were shown pictures of nature; others were shown a modern, abstract picture of straight lines and rectangles. A third group of subjects were shown a blank white wall. The patients who viewed the pictures of trees and water were significantly less anxious, and suffered less severe pain. In fact, they were able to get off the strong narcotic pain drugs the quickest. Interestingly, subjects who viewed the abstract picture actually experienced higher anxiety than those who viewed the blank wall. It kind of makes sense; the abstract picture patients were forced to view lines that do not generally occur in the natural world. Being away from the natural world produces stress.

While they are second to the real outdoors, houseplants are shown to be quite calming, too. One unique study out of Japan evaluated men who held or touched the houseplant devil's ivy for two minutes. These men were found to be calmer and more serene than the control group. The stress-activated areas of the brain (such as the amygdala) showed reduced blood flow when the men interacted with the foliage—in other words, the centers that turn on when there is stress weren't getting turned on. The study's author believed that it wasn't just devil's ivy that would have this effect; he suggested that most houseplants with soft, smooth leaves would have a similar anxiety-relieving effect.

Raised blood pressure is very common in people who have chronic anxiety. Another interesting study out of Washington State University revealed that people who enter a room full of houseplants experience clear drops in blood pressure—even if they don't directly interact with the houseplants. Another clinical trial looked at ninety patients who had hemorrhoidectomy surgeries (that's when you have painful and swollen hemorrhoid veins removed—ouch). Generally, hemorrhoids will make anyone stressed out. In this fun study, half the patients were given houseplants and flowers in their postoperative rooms. They were shown to have lower blood pressure and less pain, fatigue, and anxiety than those whose rooms did not contain plants. These patients also had higher satisfaction levels and reported that they believed the plants "brightened up the room environment and reduced my stress." The same patients reported that the hospital staff appeared more caring to them, even though both groups were treated with the same level of care. So, the plants actually led people to feel happier with the exact same care.

Electronics

In the chapter on sleep, we discussed the importance of limiting bright screens before bed. Electronics such as computers, phones, and televisions create a bright light that will suppress melatonin and make sleep difficult.

Americans use consumer electronics on an epic scale. A recent study suggests that people look at their cell phones an average of every six minutes throughout the day, with more than half admitting to checking the phone at some point while in bed. That is astounding. What's more, these electronics are all about quick-changing lights and speed. Hit a button or swipe a screen, and the information you are looking for shows up in milliseconds. It makes us feel pretty powerful. If our computer doesn't turn on in a few seconds or our cell phone isn't downloading at lighting speed, we get crazy, huffy, and maybe a bit angry, too.

A few paragraphs back, we talked about the importance of nature—plants, water scenes, calming pictures. Now contrast these images to the screen on your computer, tablet, or cell phone: it's all bright lights, pixelated images, and fast-moving animations. No wonder we are more susceptible to anxiety than we used to be. Our brains are made for nature, not touchscreens. The more time you spend using electronics, the more likely it is that you'll have anxiety in your life.

The trouble is, electronics are extraordinarily addictive. Like any other drug, you experience withdrawal symptoms when you're separated from your device. Just as cocaine users need their next fix, cell phone users are petrified of losing their phone. In fact, in a survey of Americans, seventy-three out of a hundred people will actually feel panic when they misplace their phone.

What about electronic games? For kids, electronic games are exciting; for parents, they are convenient. Your kid wants your attention at a restaurant? Just hand him an electronic game, and he'll be quiet for hours. On average, 80 to 90 percent of kids have fun with computer games. Unfortunately, kids' computer game usage has been associated with aggression and attention issues in some studies. One Iranian study of 384 male students found a 95 percent correlation between amount of electronic game usage and anxiety and depression in those youths. The younger the gamer, the more likely there will be more anxiety.

Social media is another growing concern. A United Kingdom anxiety association studied people who use social media and found that almost 50 percent of users actually get worried and have physically uncomfortable symptoms when they are cut off from Facebook. It seems people experience social media withdrawal—when they are not near it, they get anxious. About 65 percent of subjects also had sleeping problems after using various forms of social media.

So there's a strong correlation between social media and anxiety. It seems that those who use social media will experience some anxiety, but it may also be true that people who are anxious are drawn to social media. Maybe it is a way to avoid having real-life interactions. It is hard to say for sure—but either way, I strongly recommend you limit your time on social media. Maybe check it twice a day for ten minutes? This way, you stay connected, but you don't overdo it.

Also consider taking an "electronics day off" every once in a while—perhaps on a vacation day, when you can truly rest. See how you feel at the end of the day.

- No cell phone
- No TV
- No computer
- No watch or clock

By the way, if this idea makes you shudder, you may need it the most!

Deep Breathing and Meditation

We talked about the HPA axis and how cerebral thoughts will drive through to the middle of the brain and cause a full-body reaction of stress and anxiety. This is a powerful mechanism, but you have the ability to counter it. Your best weapons in this fight are mediation and deep breathing.

There's an old Buddhist riddle that I often ask my patients. Try to answer it yourself before reading the answer.

> Question: "If you truly want to be alone, where's the best place to go?"
>
> Answer: The present, because there is no one there.

I have not had one patient answer it correctly yet! The concept is fairly basic: to truly be nonanxious, you really have to be in the present moment. Anxiety is worrying about what has happened or what will happen. If you train your brain to be in the moment, it is impossible to feel anxious—the two states of being are completely incompatible.

The problem is that our untrained brain wants to run around in the past or the future. Have you ever adopted a puppy? If so, you remember that when you brought that dog home it ran around, crazily barking, chewing on things, and peeing all over the place. If you had let the dog continue on that way without instructing and disciplining it, it would have continued to run amok and eventually become very unhappy in this ruleless state. Same with children—we all need rules and guidelines to feel secure. Your brain is exactly the same way!

Your anxious brain is unhappy and undisciplined. You need meditation to discipline that unhappy puppy that is running amok. Many of my anxious patients will say, "Meditation is not for me—it just makes me more anxious." Well, I said the same thing—because I needed it the most! And likely you do, too.

For over seven thousand years, meditation has supported and calmed the human race. Out of the Buddhist tradition, we have many choices when it comes to calming our minds through relaxing breath: yoga, transcendental meditation (known as TM), Chinese qi gong, Zen Buddhism, and many others. The central idea they have in common: deeper awareness in the present moment.

The well-known neuroendocrinologist Robert Sapolsky has documented how anxiety is associated with brain cell destruction, especially in the area called the hippocampus, which is needed for balanced mood and memory. High levels of the stress hormone cortisol are known to bathe the hippocampus and actually destroy the brain tissue. As a result, people with anxiety often have shrunken hippocampi and have difficulty concentrating. As we discussed in the exercise chapter, you can regenerate brain cells by moving your body. The other proven way to regenerate your brain—and discipline it at the same time—is meditation.

Harvard researchers found that people who slowed their breathing rates through meditation for an average of forty minutes a day had positive changes in brain structure; whereas people who did not meditate had typical brain breakdown over time. The researchers used an MRI to check the brain. They found that adults had even better results than young people—maybe because an adult has more control over her thoughts. In truth, no one really understands how meditation actually benefits and rebuilds the brain—we just know it does.

As we have covered in this book, inflammation is a driver of anxiety. Well, meditation seems to help this, too. When you meditate, you encourage a nervous effect called "vagal nerve tone." Vagal nerve tone is part of your relaxation response—when you meditate, your body stops running from that bear we keep talking about. Meditation helps turn off inflammation and turn on healthy digestive function.

As far as research specifically related to anxiety, studies dating back to the early 1990s have shown how meditation training programs can effectively reduce symptoms of anxiety and panic and help maintain these reductions in patients with generalized anxiety disorder, panic, or agoraphobia (fear of being in public or crowds). But meditation isn't just for the anxious: a 2009 meta-analysis from the *Journal of Complementary and Alternative Medicine* found that mindfulness meditation can reduce stress in healthy people, too. It has also been shown to reduce ruminative thinking (thinking about things over and over—a mild type of obsessive thinking) and generalized anxiety.

Mindfulness-based cognitive therapy (MBCT) is a specific type of meditation developed by Jon Kabat Zinn. It is gaining popularity for use in parallel to psychotherapy treatment. MBCT is based on resolving feelings of stress and anxiety by processing your thoughts in a nonjudgmental way.

In order to calm anxiety, stress, and depression, start to consider your thoughts in a nonjudgmental way that allows for feelings (both emotional and physical) to be experienced and resolved in the present moment. As I said earlier, remaining in the present moment is incompatible with overwhelming feelings.

While MBCT is wonderful in theory, until recently it was unclear if this approach was actually clinically effective. In 2010, in an effort to provide a good assessment of MBCT, researchers from Boston University performed a meta-analysis. This is a study that looks at as many past studies as possible to come up with a strong conclusion. In their evaluation, the researchers analyzed thirty-nine studies totaling 1,140 subjects who worked with mind-body therapies. They called the effect of MBCT "robust," which is a significant term in medical literature. It was shown that MBCT was clearly helpful for both anxiety and depression, even when those conditions were associated with other challenges, like medical problems. The research also showed that the positive effects were long lasting. In short, MBCT works quite well for anxiety.

A Simple Meditation

While there are many wonderful and effective styles of meditation, I often teach my patients a simple one: breathe into the belly through your nose, and breathe out through your mouth. Here are the steps for a five-minute meditation. I recommend you work this into your schedule once in the morning and once in the evening every day. If you would like to increase the time as you get more comfortable, go for it!

1. Find a nice comfortable place to sit or even lie down if you like (but try not to fall asleep).

2. Set a gentle timer (like a nice chime on your cell phone) so you do not have to think about or peek at a clock to know when your time is up.

3. Relax your shoulders so they feel like jelly. Let this relaxation feeling move to your face, chest, back, hands, butt muscles, legs, and feet.

4. Gently inhale through your nose. If your nose is very stuffed up, then it is okay to breathe through your mouth. When you inhale, pretend there is a deflated balloon in your stomach. Pick a color you love for that balloon and inflate it. Be careful not to raise your chest muscles and rib cage. Put one hand on your stomach and another hand on your chest. If the chest hand is moving, you are not breathing properly. Only the hand on the stomach should be moving outward from the body on the inhale.

5. Exhale through the mouth.

Note: Create relaxed, gentle breaths—do not force them. If any thoughts come up (and they will), visualize them passing through your mind and gently moving out with the next breath. Do not worry about forcing these out—they are natural. Like an ocean wave, these thoughts will come in and go out whether we work at them or just sit back and relax. Do not judge these thoughts; just try to look at them like a passive observer.

Visit my website, *www.drpeterbongiorno.com/meditation,* to download free guided meditations.

Yoga

At five thousand years old, yoga is not quite as old as mediation practice, but it is spiritually related to meditation and deep breathing. However, yoga has a bit more movement to it and can be a powerful way to burn stress hormones. The word *yoga* comes from the Sanskrit word *yuj*, which means "yoke." Yoga is about focusing your awareness to help connect your physical, spiritual, and emotional worlds.

I think of yoga as a combination of exercise and meditation. When you breathe during yoga, you focus the mind and achieve relaxation. Like exercise, yoga is an excellent way to deepen your breathing and keep the blood flowing. Like acupuncture, which we will talk about next, yoga's aim is to clear energetic and physical blockages in the body in order to bring calm and a sense of contentment with reality. This leads to *sukha*, which is the Sanskrit word for "happiness." In Sanskrit, happiness literally means "unobstructed peace." So, yoga helps you move blocked energy to help you truly stay happy in your current situation. Even more, yoga aims to help you feel more connected to other people in the process.

Numerous studies show that you can happily and healthily change your hypothalamic pituitary adrenal axis (HPA)—your stress system function by doing yoga. Like meditation, yoga is shown to lower cortisol and balance the activity of both the parasympathetic and sympathetic nervous systems. Yoga also improves mood by maintaining proper levels of the neurotransmitter serotonin while it helps to stabilize blood sugar.

Yoga also lessens inflammation by decreasing inflammatory markers such a C-reactive protein (CRP). It also may be effective at lowering blood pressure. A significant decrease in salivary cortisol concentration was seen following a ninety-minute session of a type of yoga called Iyengar (which focuses on body alignment). Yoga will also boost the mind-calming neurotransmitter GABA. Yoga practitioners experience a significant increase in GABA levels following a sixty-minute yoga session as compared to a control group where the control volunteers calmly read magazines and fiction instead of doing yoga.

One 2005 systematic review of patients with anxiety found that yoga was an effective method of lowering stress. Another study of participants diagnosed with obsessive-compulsive disorder found that after three months, those who practiced Kundalini yoga, along with a number of other yoga techniques including mantra meditation, experienced significantly greater improvements in controlling their OCD over a control group, which practiced a basic meditation.

While yoga presents very few contraindications and practically no interaction with Western medications, it is important to start slowly and go easy if you have not tried it before, because the stretching can tax your tendons. Starting with a calm version of yoga called *hatha* might be best. If you have any physical limitations, you may want to start with private yoga instruction or tell your class yoga teacher ahead of time if you have concerns. If you are pregnant, you can still practice yoga—certain poses can be modified to accommodate pregnant bellies. Check with your physician if you have glaucoma, high blood pressure, or sciatic pain issues.

One final note: never do a yoga pose that is uncomfortable for you. As an anxious person, you might be interested in perfection—but a focus on "doing it best" will only make you more anxious. Use yoga as a way to practice and enjoy your beautiful imperfection!

Acupuncture

Acupuncture is near and dear to my heart—not only because I am an acupuncturist myself but also because when I had a serious case of anxiety with incredible insomnia, acupuncture was the first thing that helped get me to sleep. At the time, I was pretty desperate for sleep. I was offered medications that I did not want to take. I went to an acupuncturist, who listened to my story, looked at my tongue, felt my pulse, and told me quite confidently that I had something called "heart-kidney disconnect," which I did not understand at all. All I knew was that every night was a horror; as the sun went down, I dreaded the coming night, which would inevitably be filled with tossing, turning, and heart racing. If you suffer from insomnia, I don't have to tell you it is one of the worst feelings ever. That's why acupuncture was a godsend for me. It did not 100 percent fix my insomnia, but I would say that within three or four visits, I was sleeping at least half of the night. This made me functional enough to seek out the other things in this book that helped me improve overall.

The Foundation of Acupuncture: Yin and Yang

Practiced for the last three to four thousand years, acupuncture and Traditional Chinese Medicine (TCM) are based on the concept of nature. The idea is that humans come from nature, and our balance of energy (yin and yang) represents the energy of the natural world. As long as we live in harmony with the natural world, our energy should stay in balance, and we will avoid disease. Acupuncture uses fine needle insertion to access the yin and yang in our body and helps move our energy to rebalance it with nature.

Yin energy is the calm, quiet, nourishing energy of the natural world. Yang energy is the active, warm, exciting energy of nature. In the paradigm of Chinese medical thought, anxiety is often an issue of excess yang (or deficient yin). In other words, either a person has too much yang energy, or not enough yin energy to keep her centered. Most often in my practice, I see the latter—not enough yin.

Without enough yin, people become very anxious and agitated. In TCM, emotional illness is often due to accumulated anger, sorrow, and other unprocessed emotions that lead to imbalances in yin and yang. Chronic outside stress, poor food choices, lack of sleep, and inadequate movement can also unbalance the life energy force known as *qi*. As a result, "knotted qi" accumulates, and disruption of the body and mind results. Anxious people may act too "yang" (in contrast, depressed people act much more "yin").

In TCM, emotional problems often center on a particular organ. Regarding anxiety, the three organs with which I see the most associations are the kidneys, the liver, and the heart. The kidneys store our energy—like a car battery, we humans store the energy we use to move. Emotional fear causes the kidneys to deplete too fast. When the kidneys are depleted, our yin energy goes down, which makes our relative yang energy too high. That excess yang rushes up, and we end up with anxiety.

The liver is where stress is normally stored. Excess stress can cause a condition in TCM called "liver qi stagnation," which means the energy in the liver is stuck. When this energy backs up, it causes trouble in the stomach (nausea, reflux, and burping). The energy can also rise up and cause dizziness and feelings of anxiety. Some people will experience anger, hostility, or lack of motivation.

The heart houses the shen, or spirit. It encompasses thoughts, emotions, and consciousness. Your ability to react creatively, to experience joy and sorrow, come from the heart, shen. In Chinese medicine, when the shen is disturbed, anxiety, depression, and other emotional illness can result. A healthy lifestyle can help create a healthy shen.

Please note that by naming these organs, I do not imply that there is a problem with the physical organ in the Western biomedical sense—we are talking about the Chinese sense of the kidney, liver, and heart.

How Does Acupuncture Really Work?

Now that we have explored TCM and energy, let's discuss what the scientific establishment has said about acupuncture. While the full mechanism of action for acupuncture is not known, a number of studies suggest that needling the proper acupuncture points can cause the release of serotonin, norepinephrine, dopamine, beta-endorphin, and other emotionally balancing molecules called enkephalins and dynorphins. Many of these either come from or help balance the body's stress system, suggesting a direct influence on mood. Acupuncture may also influence the autonomic nervous system (the part of the nervous system that decides whether we feel stressed or calm), the immune system, inflammation, and hormones.

Does research show that acupuncture can help you with your anxiety? In 2007, a research team looked at a number of studies to figure out if acupuncture can truly help with anxiety. They found twelve good studies to support this claim; ten of these were the more stringent, randomized controlled kind. Overall, the studies found quite positive results for generalized anxiety disorder and anxiety neurosis. Auricular (ear) acupuncture was especially useful for anxiety that occurs before surgical procedures—which is a tough anxiety to treat in general. Despite these overall findings, the researchers suggested that more research would be needed to definitively prove the benefits of acupuncture.

In my experience, patients with mild to moderate anxiety do really well with calming acupuncture treatments. From time to time, those with very high anxiety may overthink the needles and find the treatment unpleasant. I try to use this fear as an opportunity—patients can calm themselves through breathing and work on negative messaging before and during their treatments. If you have anxious trepidation about getting acupuncture, tell your acupuncturist and see if he or she can help you work through it. You will be glad you did.

In my own clinic, I find clear benefits from using acupuncture in addition to or instead of conventional medicine and other natural remedies for anxiety and depression. Acupuncture can also help pharmaceutical medications to work faster and typically allows for patients to get results with lower dosages. It also supports patients who are weaning off conventional medications.

Acupuncture is exceedingly safe and does not conflict with other treatments, natural remedies, psychological care, or drugs. It is even safe for pregnant women and does not interfere with breast-feeding. Large-scale studies have reviewed millions of treatments and have found almost no risk. For example, one 2009 survey looked at almost 230,000 acupuncture patients and found only three patients had sustained an injury from treatment, and none of these were life-threatening.

Resources for good acupuncturists are listed in appendix II.

Massage

Along with acupuncture, therapeutic massage is among the most ancient of healthcare practices. Hippocrates told his students that every physician must be acquainted with "rubbing," for he knew the importance of therapeutic touch and the value of moving the body and increasing circulation. Massage helps move the lymph tissue, too—this helps the body detoxify. It will also help loosen tense muscles and relax the nervous system.

Studies from the mid-1990s show that massage increases calm and lowers levels of the stress hormone cortisol by 30 percent. At the same time, it increases levels of the feel-good neurotransmitters dopamine and serotonin by about the same amount.

Some studies have shown massage to be effective in reducing both targeted anxiety (associated with a specific event) and general anxiety, as well as blood pressure and heart rate, pain, and depression. One literature review even suggested massage might be as good as psychotherapy for anxiety states. Looking at thirty-seven randomized, controlled trials on massage, this review found that, on average, the massage therapy participants experienced a reduction in anxiety of at least 77 percent as compared to controls. Comparatively, psychotherapy for these conditions has been shown to have a 79 percent benefit rate over untreated patients. I vote to use both together for even better results.

Before I started regular massage treatments, I thought I would never get comfortable with the idea of a massage. I didn't like the idea of being that vulnerable. Now, I find massage to be a wonderful therapeutic experience that is profoundly relaxing—and I can't go often enough! If you are anxious about massage, talk to your massage therapist and let him know.

Checklist for Healthy Mind-Body

- ❏ Get adequate sunlight (consider a light box, if needed)
- ❏ Get out into nature
- ❏ Avoid electronics when possible
- ❏ Breathing and meditation work
- ❏ Choose at least one mind-body therapy:
    - ❏ Yoga
    - ❏ Acupuncture
    - ❏ Massage

supplements

Case: Marissa

When I first met Marissa, she was almost twenty-one years old. Her parents divorced when she was nineteen and still in college. Around the same time, a close friend passed away while traveling as a passenger in the car of a drunk driver. Soon after these two life-changing events, Marissa started getting anxiety—which she had never experienced before. It took the form of performance anxiety, coming on in situations like taking a test or speaking in front of groups of people. She started to feel dizzy at parties and social gatherings. Her sleep also started to suffer.

For about one year, Marissa bounced from one anxiety pill to another. First, her primary care doctor gave her Xanax for daytime use. This did not seem to help, so she was prescribed Klonopin in the evenings as her sleep worsened. When experienced blurred vision and hand and foot swelling, the medications were stopped after four months. Then she tried the "gentler" Ativan, which also did not help and caused more blurry vision and constipation.

Marissa's doctor decided to switch gears and try the selective serotonin reuptake inhibitor (SSRI) class of drugs. First up was Lexapro. After four weeks, Lexapro did seem to bring anxiety down, but the nausea was over the top. She switched to Zoloft, which worked less well, and brought on a similar nausea that did not wane after eight weeks.

Nauseated and frustrated, Marissa was referred to me by a friend whose mom had worked with me for digestive problems a few years earlier. Marissa explained her story and how the SSRI drugs were helpful, but the side effects were debilitating.

After we covered the basics (diet, lifestyle, some basic blood tests), I realized that Marissa had a tremendous stressor that put her neurotransmitters out of whack. My thought here was simple: Marissa did not do well on benzodiazepines (Xanax, Ativan), but did well on SSRI medications (Lexapro, Zoloft). SSRIs stop serotonin from being broken down by poisoning enzyme systems in the brain. Like many of my patients, Marissa was too sensitive to take them.

So why not try a gentler, more natural form? I gave Marissa some 5-HTP, a special form of tryptophan that the brain absorbs easily. Tryptophan can help naturally support the serotonin system, without the side effects. Marissa started at 50 mg twice a day. I gave her a gentle multiple vitamin full of B vitamins (cofactors that help make serotonin), as well as some fish oil and probiotics.

Within one week, Marissa was feeling about 50 percent better. We raised the tryptophan dosage to 100 mg twice a day, and within three weeks, she felt 100 percent better, without any side effects. We also continued to work on her diet and lifestyle, and I sent her to a specialized therapist to help with both the grief of losing her family structure, and the grief of tragically losing a close friend.

The above case shows us how gentle natural remedies can help bring people into balance and can be more potent and offer fewer side effects than their pharmaceutical counterparts. However, the many supplements we are about to talk about are one part of the big picture. Remember the stool illustration from the introduction? Supplements are one leg. One leg by itself can't hold you up completely, but used in conjunction with a full naturopathic program, supplements can be hugely effective. I want to be clear: supplementation by itself is *not* the solution to your anxiety. "Supplements" are just that: they *supplement* your healthy lifestyle, diet, and thoughts. Many of my first-time patients who have seen other well-meaning practitioners come to me with a big bag of supplements that they take every day—yet they still do not feel better. This is a common scenario I do not want to see for you.

My hope is that you get to a place where you do not believe you need anything from a bottle, whether it is a drug or a supplement. That will require you to fully absorb the first seven chapters of this book, and do the best you can to truly improve your thoughts, sleep, exercise, diet, and mind-body work. If we can pick the right couple of supplements to help you along, then that is a good thing that will get you there even faster.

We have already talked about a number of supplements that help with sleep, digestion, and nutrient and hormone balance. Here, we will run through all the other helpful anxiety-busting supplements. Remember, you can't take them all—so read closely and identify the ones that might be most specifically helpful for your particular needs.

When it comes to supplements, it's best to start with the basics. For almost any condition, there are three supplements I like to use: a multiple vitamin, a fish oil, and a probiotic. The triumvirate for basic health, I call them the "Three U Need." These are also found at *www.3UNeed.com.*

While there may be specific supplements I might use as individual issues pop up, these are the three I take regularly for my overall health. Let's go through each of them briefly and talk about how they can be a fantastic support for you as you beat anxiety.

Multiple Vitamin

Multiple vitamins are basically a shotgun approach to nutritional supplementation. We know that a number of vitamins and minerals are useful for basic processes in our body. A multiple vitamin brings them all together and gives you some of each.

But do you really need a multiple? And will it help your anxiety? Well, you know that when your nutrients are low, your mood goes south. The standard American diet that many of us use to keep our bodies nourished is woefully low in vegetables and whole foods. As a result, you become deficient in the things you really need. For example, quality protein breaks down into amino acids. Amino acids like tryptophan are the building blocks of neurotransmitters—our molecules of emotion. Without protein, our neurotransmitter levels suffer.

You might say, "That doesn't apply to me. I eat a very healthy diet." Maybe you do. Consider this: the most complete studies on the subject show that even people who think they eat a healthy diet are in trouble. The American Dietetic Association reviewed seventy dietary analyses of over twenty different diets from a cross section of people, ranging from elite athletes (who had phenomenally healthy food intake) to nonexercisers who ate poorly. What was shown was that no diet, even among the people who ate well, contained 100 percent of the recommended daily allowance (RDA) of needed nutrients. And guess what? The athletes were the most deficient of all.

Researchers out of Australia gave fifty healthy men (aged fifty to seventy) either a multiple vitamin or a placebo. They found that the men who took the vitamin had lower stress and more energy. As a result, they got more done. Studies out of the United Kingdom also showed that a good multiple vitamin helped mild mood problems and was associated with lower stress and increased energy.

How to Dose a Multiple Vitamin

I always tell my patients to pick a good quality multiple vitamin in capsule form (which means it has powder in it—rather than a tablet, which is hard and typically more difficult for the body to break down). The average dose for a quality capsule is three to six per day. I know that sounds like a lot, but it is usually necessary in the beginning—after all, you need to replace lost nutrients from years of anxiety. After a few months you can bring the dose down to half, and few months later to a quarter (if your whole food intake is high).

The 2013 U.S. Preventive Services Task Force series study shows no side effects or toxicity associated with multiple vitamins. Trials of over 27,000 people suggest less cancer in people who take a multivitamin.

Fish Oil

Fish oil contains fatty acids that help make high-quality membranes for every cell in your body. Healthy membranes mean good communication, ability to get rid of toxins, and lower inflammation in the body. Fish oil also contains essential fatty acids we need for a healthy nervous system. "Essential" means your body can't make them by itself—so if you are not taking enough in, there's no way to really keep optimal mood and sense of well-being. For your nervous system, fish oil helps make brain-derived neurotrophic factor (BDNF) and nerve growth factor (NGF). Both of these are responsible for growth and repair, and it is hard to recover from anxiety without these working well. Finally, fish oil has been shown to be a direct support and benefit for your adrenal glands. Those are the glands at the top of the kidneys that get way overused when you get stressed out.

People with anxiety have been shown to have quite low levels of the essential fatty acids eicosapentaenoic acid (EPA) and docosahexaenoic acid (DHA)—the main components of fish oil. In fact, it has been shown that EPA and DHA levels are directly correlated with anxiety. Scans of people with anxiety found that low levels of DHA mess up the use of sugars in the brain—when it can't get or use sugar, it thinks it's starving, and the primitive stress response kicks into gear. In this state, it is shown that people are not able to make decisions or resolve problems easily. Low DHA also allows parts of the brain called the anterior cingulate gyrus and prefrontal cortex to get too active and contribute to mood problems. So is there evidence that fish oil really helps anxiety and mood? Absolutely. In fact, I think it should be put in the water here in New York City where I practice. (Just kidding, I don't think oil and water really mixes well.)

Medical school is crazy stressful: constant tests, friends failing out, new activities you do not feel comfortable doing or seeing, and very little sleep. A twelve-week study of stressed-out medical students showed that those who took a half-teaspoon of fish oil had 14 percent less inflammation in their body, and a 20 percent decrease in symptoms of anxiety over those who took a placebo. That is a pretty small amount of fish oil for a pretty short period of time— if researchers had given the students a full teaspoon as I do with my patients, the benefits would have been even stronger. (It is not uncommon in research to see students underdose natural supplements. It seems that researchers are afraid of supplements, but drug toxicity is less of a concern. Although it seems far-fetched, it is not out of the realm of possibility that pharmaceutical companies may indirectly fund these studies. Low dosages yield more negative studies that make supplements look bad, so the media can carry the message that "fish oil doesn't work.")

Given how it supports the brain and nervous system, it is not surprising that fish oil also benefits patients with depression, schizophrenia, and those who fail to respond to selective serotonin reuptake inhibitors (SSRIs) for depression.

How to Dose Fish Oil

Typically, I recommend about 3 or 4 grams of fish oil a day, measuring around 900 mg of EPA and 800 mg of DHA. If your fish oil label doesn't give you these numbers, buy another one that does. Fish oil comes in capsules or liquid. While most people shy away from the liquid, it is good to remember that your grandmother probably used it that way, so there must be some benefit to it.

Some people experience burping with fish oil. Try taking it with food and without food, and see what works best for you. My patients have taught me that you can refrigerate the capsules and take while cold to reduce the burpiness. If burping is a real problem, try an enteric coated capsule, which opens up later in the digestive tract to avoid stomach reflux. Unfortunately, our stewardship of the seas has become very poor, so no corner of the ocean is without toxins. As a result, you need to look for "molecularly distilled" fish oil, which has gone through a process that eliminates 100 percent of toxins like mercury and dioxins.

Fish oil is extremely safe, but if you are taking medications that change the clotting in your blood (sometimes called blood thinners), it is best to check with your physician before using fish oil. Recently, there were media reports that fish oil causes prostate cancer. Several of my male patients contacted me about the news. I found the reports odd because many research studies suggest that fish oil *prevents* certain cancers, including prostate cancer. This study was published in a well-respected journal, the *Journal of the National Institute of Cancer*, which is part of the National Institutes of Health. I looked at this study closely and found that it was designed to test vitamin E, not fish oil supplements. The study did not track supplements at all—instead, researchers used surrogate markers of fish oil at two paltry time points over six years and extrapolated the rest. In this case, "extrapolated" is a fancy word for "kind of made up based on almost no information." If I had handed in an experiment and writeup like this in my high school science class, I would have failed. That this study was published in a prestigious journal and passed off to the public as factual is a testament to medical establishment's bias against natural medicine. Interestingly, a very unpublicized recent *British Medical Journal* analysis of twenty-one studies of over one million people showed that fish oil intake and omega-3 fat intake reduced breast cancer occurrence significantly. Amazing how the media kind of missed that one!

Food Sources of Fish Oil

Can you guess where to find fish oil? It's Grant's Tomb. Oh wait, that's another joke . . . anyway, it's fish! Some studies suggest that eating the fish itself might be the best way to absorb the oil. Do your best—I find it hard to eat enough fish, so I also use a supplement.

Small fish such as anchovies, herring, and sardines are fine omega-3 sources. Larger fish such as tuna, shark, swordfish, mackerel, and salmon are very good, but some may be contaminated with mercury and harmful pesticides. Please find the fish-mercury content listing in chapter 5. You might be surprised to learn that chicken, eggs, and beef can actually be reasonable sources of omega-3 fatty acids—but only if the animal was grass-fed.

What about Vegan Oils for Vegetarians?

While vegan oils like flax and sesame oil may have some benefit, they need to be converted to EPA in the body. Unfortunately for many people with standing mood-disorder issues, the enzyme that does this is often not functioning well. As a result, the vegetarian oils may not fully support the brain and nervous system the way fish oil can. I recommend fish oil if are you willing. If this is not possible for you for ethical reasons, you might consider algae-derived essential fats, flax oil, or rapeseed oil. The best sources of vegan omega-3 fats are found in these oils, as well as walnuts and tofu.

Probiotics

We talked about the importance of the "healthy germs" in your digestive tract, known as your microbiome, in the food section of chapter 5. If you need to refresh about this fascinating topic, please go back to the food section.

Now we are going to discuss the supplements commonly called probiotics. These are designed to support your microbiome and can help lower anxiety. In animal studies, anxiety-prone mice that were given probiotics were more chilled out than ones that were not.

These chilled-out mice had lower levels of corticosterone, the mouse version of our human stress hormone cortisol. Another study found that putting the germs from a stressed mouse into a nonstressed mouse showed that the nonstressed animal became stressed out. By the way, this poop-swapping procedure is called a "fecal transplant" (now you can say "eeeeewww") and can potentially be used for a number of conditions, including ulcerative colitis, a serious inflammatory disease of the colon.

While there are just a few human studies on probiotics and mood, these are quite promising for anxiety sufferers. In healthy, nonanxious and nondepressed people, strains of the probiotic *lactobacillus* and *bifidobacterium* administered for just thirty days lowered psychological distress and depression, decreased anger and hostility, lessened anxiety, and improved problem solving, compared to the placebo group. In another study, patients with chronic fatigue who were given lactobacillus for sixty days also found far fewer anxiety symptoms than the placebo group.

Dosage of Probiotics

Different studies have used varying strains and dosages of probiotics. Most studies use lactobacillus and bifidus, so in my practice, I recommend these, dosed at 4 billon organisms three times a day. I will dose significantly higher if a patient is taking, or has a long history of taking, antibiotics. While very safe, probiotics may be contraindicated in some patients who have bleeding of the intestines. Since quality varies wildly, please purchase a probiotic from a reputable manufacturer, for poorly made probiotics have been shown to be ineffective and also can contain dangerous bacteria, like *E. coli.*

Please see *www.3UNeed.com* for more information about high-quality multiple vitamins, fish oil supplements, and probiotics.

Minerals

We just discussed the pillars of a good supplement regimen: a multiple vitamin, a fish oil, and a probiotic. Now we are going to talk about a few other supplements that are also excellent supports for patients with anxiety. These do not directly adjust mood like the third-line options we will discuss in a little bit, but they are still designed to give support to your basic physiology.

B Vitamins: B3, B6, B12, Folate, and Inositol

B vitamins are incredibly important if you are stressed out. Stress burns through these vitamins, and yet they are greatly needed to keep our body healthy during stress. B vitamins play an important role in neurotransmitter production and homocysteine regulation (a sign of inflammation discussed in appendix I), both of which correlate with mood. Low levels of B vitamins correlate with higher anxiety symptoms in large epidemiologic studies. Let's talk a little more about these wonderful B vitamins.

Vitamin B3

Known for its effectiveness as a treatment for anxiety conditions on its own, vitamin B3 (niacinamide) helps mood in two ways. One, it stops the liver's breakdown of tryptophan, the amino acid needed for your body to produce anxiety-relieving serotonin. In fact, sometimes I dose 500 mg of B3 with tryptophan if patients are having trouble staying asleep. Two, B3 activates the conversion of tryptophan to 5-HTP. Vitamin B3 supplementation prevented development of anxiety in baby animals that were exposed to low oxygen around the time of birth when compared to a placebo group.

Vitamin B6

Vitamin B6 (pyridoxine) is a main cofactor in the conversion of tryptophan to serotonin. Vitamin B6 deficiency contributes to low mood. Birth control pills are known to deplete vitamin B6. Research from the early 1980s showed that supplementation with 40 mg per day of B6 helped both anxiety and depression in women who took vitamin-depleting birth control. Other studies supplementing vitamin B6 found modest anxiety benefit in anxious females with premenstrual disorder who were prescribed 200 mg of magnesium along with 50 mg of vitamin B6.

Vitamin B12

Vitamin B12 (methylcobalamin) is a key player in the synthesis of serotonin. There is some evidence that people with depression respond better to treatment if they have higher levels of vitamin B12. Anecdotal reports from Dr. Alan Gaby, a nutrient teacher of mine and expert on the subject of vitamins, suggest that weekly intramuscular administration of vitamin B12 may improve unexplained anxiety in patients with normal serum vitamin B12. I have also used sublingual lozenges with good results.

Folic Acid (Folate)

The word *folate* comes from the Latin word "folium," which means leaf—and the best source of folic acid is in leafy greens. Depletion of folic acid can happen with chronic medication or birth control use, chronic alcohol intake, and not eating enough leafy greens. Low folate makes it harder for serotonin-boosting drugs to work their best, and folate is also needed to help dopamine, serotonin, and epinephrine uptake. Proper amounts of folate also help keep homocysteine levels under control. I talk more about homocysteine's relationship to anxiety in appendix I.

Inositol

A lightly sweet plant-derived powder, inositol is not a true B vitamin, but it is typically incorporated with the Bs. In 1996, one inositol study used about 18 grams a day for both obsessive-compulsive issues and panic disorder. Another follow-up work for patients with panic had twenty patients taking the same dose and compared their results to the drug Luvox (an SSRI-type medication). The study found that panic attacks were reduced by four episodes on average in the inositol patients. I would love to see more studies on inositol.

B Complex

Usually, B vitamins are not given alone but in combination. This is how I typically use them in my clinic, especially for anxious patients who are combatting regular daily stress. One research study on B vitamins gave sixty stressed out employees a B complex for three months. At the end of the study, the B complex group had much lower "personal strain and a reduction in confusion and depressed/dejected mood." Basically, B complex vitamins helped these people hold up under chronic daily stress. A University of Miami trial evaluated a B complex supplement in sixty adult depressed patients for sixty days. There were significant improvements in both depressive and anxiety symptoms. While this study and its author were supported by the company that made the vitamins, the results are consistent with what we know from other works.

B Complex, Folate, and Inositol Dosage

I recommend using a B complex, which includes daily amounts of vitamins B1 (thiamine 100 mg), B2 (riboflavin 25 mg), B3 (niacinamide 75 mg), B5 (pantothenic acid 200 mg), B6 (pyridoxal 5'-phosphate 15 mg), and B12 (methylcobalamin 500 mcg). It typically will also include some folate (L-methylfolate 400 mcg). Please note the fancy forms of these—they are high quality and more well utilized by the body. These dosages are also higher than typically given in studies, but I find my anxious patients burn through them pretty quickly. Once anxiety is under control, lower doses can be used for maintenance.

Sometimes adding extra amounts of single B vitamins in certain cases is useful, too. For instance, taking 100 mg of B3 several times daily with meals may enhance the effectiveness of supplemental tryptophan doses, which is useful for both anxiety and depression. Depending on the individual case, I will often dose extra sublingual B12 (up to 5000 mcg per day) and folate (up to 2 mg total). Additionally, I may also consider adding a powdered inositol if there is a strong anxiety, obsessive-compulsive, or panic picture (up to 18 grams a day).

B Vitamins, Folic Acid, and Inositol Toxicity

B vitamins are water-soluble and do not accumulate in the body, so toxicity is very unlikely. I have never seen it in my practice. It should be noted that high doses of vitamin B6 (more than 200 mg a day) may cause a reversible tingling or neuropathy in the hands and feet, along with fatigue. Do not use more than 100 mg per day of B6 to be safe. Folic acid forms should not be combined with methotrexate when used to treat cancer (for it blocks the ability of the drug to kill cancer cells), but should be used with methotrexate when treating rheumatoid arthritis. If you take methotrexate, ask your doctor about this. Inositol seems to have no toxicity, but I have seen two patients have minor stomach discomfort that went away once inositol was stopped.

Food Sources of B Vitamins, Folic Acid, and Inositol

Overall, the best sources for most B vitamins, and vitamins in general, are leafy green vegetables like kale, spinach, and chard. Top vitamin B6 sources include bell peppers, spinach, and turnip greens. Top sources of vitamin B3 include chicken, turkey, and beef. The best vegetable sources include peas, sunflower seeds, and avocados. Vitamin B12 is found in high levels in snapper and calf's liver. Vegetarian food sources have significantly lower available B12; these are kelp, algaes (like blue-green algae), and brewer's yeast. Methylfolate is found in spinach, asparagus, romaine lettuce, turnip greens, collard greens, and many more vegetables and beans. Some good inositol sources include most vegetables, nuts, and wheat germ.

Magnesium

If I had to pick a favorite supplement, it might be magnesium. Great for the heart and blood vessels, it is relaxing to both your muscles and your nervous system. It has been my ally to balance anxiety for years.

Magnesium deficiency is rampant, because we are processing our foods and stripping it away in that process. Note that any food with processed flour in it (like all white breads, bagels, cookies . . .) have a paltry 16 percent of their mineral and magnesium content left! As we learned in the food section of this book, simple carbs strip magnesium from the body. Furthermore, filtration will strip away any natural mineral content from water sources. Low levels of magnesium will encourage inflammation in your body and make it harder for your brain to maintain neurotransmitter levels, which need magnesium as a cofactor. A Norwegian research group looked at almost six thousand people aged forty-six to seventy-four years and found correlation between low intake of magnesium and high levels of anxiety and depression.

Magnesium Dosage and Toxicity

In my clinic, 250 mg twice a day is a typical dose. Some people may need up to 800 mg total per day. I like to use magnesium glycinate or taurate forms. Also, Epsom salt baths are a great form of magnesium; Epsom salt is magnesium sulphate, and it is easily absorbed through the skin into the body, especially for relaxation of muscles. Magnesium is quite nontoxic. Two concerns to keep in mind: if your stool gets a bit loose, you may need to back off on the magnesium dosage. Also, if you have any kidney concerns, magnesium may not be appropriate, so talk to your doctor.

Take a Magnesium Bath

Try one or two cups of Epsom salt in a bath at night for extra calming. Add a few drops of lavender essential oil to the bath for even more relaxation.

Food Sources of Magnesium

Mineral water is a great magnesium source. It may be the reason that the French, who drink large quantities of mineral water, have low rates of heart disease. Other magnesium sources include blackstrap molasses, summer squash, spinach, halibut, turnip greens, and seeds (pumpkin, sunflower, and flax).

Chromium

As we talked about in chapter 5, when blood sugar is all over the place, anxiety skyrockets. This is because low and fluctuating blood sugar causes an anxiety response from the brain. Chromium is a trace mineral that forms the center of a molecule called glucose tolerance factor (GTF). GTF carries blood sugar around the body and helps insulin properly take sugar crystals out of the blood and place them into your body cells where they belong. Chromium also aids proper serotonin activity.

Chromium Dosage

With no known side effects at the standard dosage of 200 mcg per day, chromium is a reasonable choice for any anxious patient showing challenges with blood sugar, whether it's chronically low, fluctuating, or high. For ongoing blood sugar problems, I will give 200 mcg three times a day with meals.

Food Sources of Chromium

Brewer's yeast is one of my favorite chromium sources. You can also get it from onions, tomatoes, and romaine lettuce. Liver is a good source, too, but make sure it comes from animals that are naturally raised in order to avoid extra toxins stored in the liver.

Selenium

Selenium is another trace mineral that helps the body maintain its own powerful antioxidants. Selenium is known to help prevent cancer, produce neurotransmitters, and support the conversion of the thyroid hormone thyroxine (T4) to its more active form, triiodothyronine (T3). When patients are given selenium in clinical trials, anxiety goes down.

Selenium Dosage and Toxicity

Usually, for patients with anxiety who have issues converting T4 to T3, I recommend 100 to 200 mcg of selenium a day. Toxicity can cause some dermatitis, hair issues, and nail brittleness. While these occur at very high doses, I recommend not taking more than 400 mcg a day.

Food Sources of Selenium

Best sources of selenium include meat, fish, Brazil nuts, and garlic.

Lithium

Lithium is a mineral I first heard about when Nirvana came out with the song "Lithium" in 1991. I was trying to make it in a rock band at the time, so anything Nirvana did was exciting to me. Kurt Cobain was actually writing about the drug form lithium carbonate used for bipolar disorder, but we are going to talk about the natural supplement lithium and its use for anxiety.

Lithium is known to make people feel good. Higher levels of natural lithium in the environment and water correlate with lower levels of suicide. Lithium spring water areas in Saratoga, New York, were used by the Iroquois for healing and well-being. In fact, the soda drink 7-Up contained a lithium supplement until 1950 (and, as an aside, you may not know that Coca-Cola used to have a little cocaine in it—not the healthiest way to give people a lift).

Lithium seems to help the brain in numerous ways: it protects nerve cells from damage and helps new ones grow by supporting levels of the super-brain repair molecule brain-derived neurotropic factor (BDNF). Exercise, probiotics, and fish oil can also increase BDNF, which is low in people with anxiety. Lithium may also increase levels of the protective fatty acid DHA in the brain. In fact, patients treated with lithium seem to have significantly lower rates of Alzheimer's disease.

Lithium also helps promote oxytocin in the body. Oxytocin is an important feel-good neurotransmitter that is secreted in high levels when you get a massage or relax and eat a nice meal with friends. People who typically feel lonely have lower rates of oxytocin. Lithium also seems to support increased levels of gamma-aminobutyric acid (GABA) in the brain. GABA is a calming neurotransmitter that is often low in anxious people. Finally, some cell culture research has shown that lithium can increase antioxidant levels in the brain, too. Wow—this supplement can take on anxiety from a number of angles.

A number of rat studies have shown that lithium will raise oxytocin. In one small study, twenty long-term marijuana smokers were given 500 mg of the drug lithium carbonate twice daily for seven days. Three months later, most of these smokers were getting high less often—and some gave up the habit completely. The study's authors mentioned those who stopped completely had greater levels of happiness than those who just smoked less.

I usually recommend supplemental lithium, which is called lithium orotate. This type of lithium gets into the brain easier than the drug. As a result, you can take much less, which takes less of a toll on the body and has fewer side effects, too. While lithium carbonate is dosed around 180 mg a day, lithium orotate can have an effect at 5 mg. Unfortunately, there are no formal studies on supplemental lithium. Oftentimes, natural supplements are not studied because there is no money to be made on substances you cannot patent and mark up for a profit. But this doesn't mean we shouldn't study them for the greater good of the public. Anyway, I welcome future studies on supplemental lithium orotate.

Lithium Orotate Dosage and Toxicity

Lithium orotate is used at doses of 5 mg to 20 mg a day. While these supplemental doses show no toxicity, we do know that high doses of the drug form can be problematic, and this is theoretically possible with the supplement as well. The drug is known to cause dull personality, blunting of emotions, memory loss, tremors, and weight gain. Long-term, high-dosage use of the drug can also mess up the kidneys and thyroid. While I have never seen or read of these issues with the supplement form of lithium, be cautious and use under direction of a knowledgeable practitioner. There are hair analysis tests and blood tests that can detect levels of lithium in the body (see appendix I)—I prefer to perform these tests before giving the supplement and then again while the patient is taking the supplement. Adequate levels of vitamin A and vitamin E may help protect the body from too much lithium.

Food Sources of Lithium
Thyme may contain the highest levels of natural lithium, and whole grains and green vegetables contain trace amounts. In some cultures, people keep thyme-infused oil on the table to add to food. This might be a nice way to try it at home.

Zinc

Zinc is another important trace mineral that you need in the right amounts for good mood. When levels of zinc are low, anxiety issues are more likely. Like lithium, zinc can help increase BDNF. We also know that you need zinc in order to make GABA, the calming neurotransmitter. When zinc is low in relationship to copper levels in the body, anxiety is even more likely (see appendix I).

Zinc Dosage and Toxicity
Typical zinc dosage is 15 mg a day. If zinc stores are very low, then 30 mg a day would be a good start for two months, after which you can lower to 15 mg. Zinc is best taken with food in order to avoid nausea.

Food Sources of Zinc
Animal sources top the list when it comes to zinc: lamb, turkey, beef, and lobster, among others. Pumpkin seed is the best vegetarian source and one of my favorites—I like them raw in order to get healthy oils, too. For men, pumpkin seed is great for prostate health.

Amino Acids

Amino acid supplementation holds an important place in anxiety treatment, for amino acids are the direct building blocks for neurotransmitters. I have seen time and time again how properly prescribed amino acids can help anxious patients achieve mood balance in order to move forward with life.

Gamma Amino-Butyric Acid (GABA) and Phenibut

As the premier calming neurotransmitter, GABA is needed for calm. Supplemental GABA is basically like a very mild benzodiazepine drug (like Xanax or Ativan). (Please note that it is not as powerful as these drugs, and the side effects are not as likely either!) GABA helps open up nerve cells to slow nerve firing when it's too fast—this helps calm the brain and your anxiety.

Unfortunately, there isn't a lot of research on GABA. The few existing studies do suggest it can help. One study prescribed 100 mg of GABA or placebo to sixty-three adults. In the people taking GABA, brain EEG studies showed more balanced alpha waves. Alpha waves are produced when the brain is relaxed and feeling peaceful. Most often, you see these waves during sleep and meditation. A second study showed alpha-enhancing activity from supplemental GABA. And when people with fear of heights were given the GABA, the GABA normalized body functions, even while they were scared—something that did not happen with placebo.

Phenibut is a form of GABA known as beta-phenyl-gamma-amino-butyric acid. This lesser-known but more highly concentrated form of GABA is used as a prescription drug in countries like Russia. It is available over the counter in the US. While there isn't much published clinical research on phenibut, there are a few decades of use and basic research that suggests strong benefit.

GABA and Phenibut Dosage and Toxicity

GABA is useful for calming during the day, as a sleep aid, and for staying sleep (when you can't get yourself into that alpha state we talked about above). There is some research that suggests the reason GABA works well for some and not others is that GABA is a molecule that is hard to get into the brain unless both the gut and the brain barriers are a little leaky. Try GABA and see if it helps you calm down. For sensitive individuals, I often recommend starting with 250 mg, going up to 750 mg without food. Do not take more than 1,000 mg in a four-hour window, or 3,000 mg within a twenty-four-hour period. Wait a half hour and see if you feel calmer. If this doesn't help, try phenibut at a dose of 300 mg. If no benefit, take up to 900 mg of phenibut when you feel you need it for either extreme anxiety or sleeping problems.

I consider GABA to be quite safe for long-term use over a few months. Phenibut is more of a concern for me, so I recommend patients take it only as needed and not on a regular basis (more than a week or two without a break). Because it is stronger, it can become addictive, like antianxiety medications. Also remember that when these supplements work, they do not "fix" the causes of anxiety. That is why the topics in the rest of this book are so important to master.

Food Sources of GABA

GABA is at highest levels in green, black, and oolong teas. This could be why sitting for four o'clock tea can be so relaxing. Fermented foods such as kim qi and yogurt contain GABA, as do oats.

Glycine

Like GABA, glycine calms nerves while decreasing release of epinephrine in the brain. It is the simplest amino acid from a structural standpoint, but may be the most useful for anxiety and panic. Two small, double-blind, placebo-controlled studies of fourteen and sixteen healthy patients exposed to loud sounds found that high doses of glycine calmed the brain's cortex (the place we do our thinking) and decreased reaction to the sound. Since the cortex is the place where it all starts (see figure 2.1, p. 10), this is an important supplement in my anxiety toolbox. In my New York practice, when a patient tells me she "jumps every time an ambulance comes by," I know glycine will be helpful.

Glycine Dosage and Toxicity

A good glycine schedule is one teaspoon (about 5 grams) of powder in a little water up to four times a day. It is a sweet and pleasant-tasting powder. My teacher Dr. Bill Mitchell taught us to add a dropperful (about 30 drops) of passionflower to the mixture for added calming benefit. Take it up to four times a day for general anxiety, or take a half hour before an expected stressful event. While glycine has no known toxicity, those with kidney or liver disease should check with their doctors before adding relatively high doses of any amino acid.

Lysine and Arginine

I consider lysine and arginine to be brothers of sorts, for I like to use them together. Lysine lowers the activity of the anxiety-producing part of the brain called the amygdala, while adjusting serotonin in such a way that it helps decrease digestive symptoms when they are caused by stress. Arginine calms the hypothalamus, so the stress system calms down and the stress hormone cortisol stays low.

Studies of using lysine and arginine for anxiety have both shown benefits. In the first, men with high anxiety levels were given 3 grams a day of each, or placebo, for ten days. The men taking the supplements were more able to handle the stress of public speaking, while the placebo had no effect. A second evaluation of 108 anxious people given 2.6 grams of lysine and arginine per day found lower salivary cortisol in men, but not in women. While I am not clear why this effect was only found in men, we do know that women tend to run higher levels of cortisol; it's possible that this study was not run long enough to see women's levels of cortisol decrease. More importantly, though, the study did show that both men and women experienced greatly lowered feelings of fear, tension, and apprehension.

Lysine and Arginine Dosage and Toxicity

Both are dosed at 2 to 3 grams each, twice a day, taken away from food. They are known to be safe in the long term. Some literature suggests that arginine may exacerbate herpetic sores if present. Lysine may actually help herpes sores, and is used as a natural treatment for them.

N-Acetyl-Cysteine (NAC)

N-acetyl-cysteine is a potent generator of the master body antioxidant glutathione. It is also well known in emergency care circles as the go-to remedy for liver toxicity. NAC has been studied in many clinical trials for use with obsessive-compulsive disorder, hair pulling (known as trichotillomania), and gambling addiction. NAC has also been successfully used in children and adolescents with autism, as well as in adults with depression and bipolar disorder. I also use NAC for patients who have chronic sinusitis issues, for it helps clear mucous from the nose and respiratory tract. I see many people who have their nose stuff up when they are anxious, and NAC is perfect for them.

N-Acetyl-Cysteine Dosage and Toxicity

Typical dosages of NAC are 500–600 mg two or three times a day away from food. NAC is non-toxic. One study of young people with a nail-biting habit did report headaches, agitation, withdrawal, and some aggression. Avoid if taking chemotherapy.

Food Sources of N-Acetyl-Cysteine

While there are no direct food sources of NAC, cysteine is a precursor of NAC, and is found in high-protein foods like meat, tofu, eggs, and dairy products.

Phosphatidylserine (PS)

Nerve cell membranes are made of phosphatidylserine and fatty acids. As a prime membrane component, PS is responsible for cell-to-cell communication and regulation of nutrients and toxins. It also plays a role in inflammatory response. In regards to anxiety, PS can help lower your stress hormone cortisol.

Trials where 800 mg of PS was given to healthy men showed a potent lowering of cortisol when exposed to exercise stressors. Researchers interested in combining the anxiety-supporting power of PS with omega-3 fats gave sixty healthy men either 300 mg of an omega-rich PS supplement or a placebo for three months. PS and the omega fats had stress-reducing effects for those subjects who had chronically high stress. This was impressive, given that this was pretty low dose of PS and omega fats. But the other volunteers who were not chronically stressed out were not affected. This suggests that the treatment worked in an adaptogenic fashion—natural adaptogens help your body raise stress chemical levels when they are too low and lower the levels when they are too high.

Phosphatidylserine Dosage and Toxicity

I usually recommend 200 to 300 mg of PS up to three times a day, in between meals. Like glycine or GABA, PS can be especially useful before stressful events. I will typically recommend phosphatidylserine for the highly stressed or depressed person who is under great physical stress and who has high cortisol and poor memory. Also, phosphatidylserine may work best when taken in conjunction with essential fatty acids. No toxicity has been reported in studies of PS.

Food Sources of Phosphatidylserine
PS amounts are highest in herring, mackerel, liver, chicken liver, white beans, and clams.

Taurine

Taurine is made from the amino acid cysteine with the help of vitamin B6. It supports glycine and GABA levels, and thereby helps calm the brain and nervous system. It can also detoxify the brain of glutamate, an excitatory amino acid that promotes anxiety. It is also a known anticlotting factor. While some animal studies show taurine as an anxiety buster, no human studies have yet confirmed this. Nevertheless, I have seen compelling anecdotal evidence that taurine is effective at controlling anxiety.

Taurine Dosage and Toxicity
Taurine is usually dosed about 500 mg up to three times daily. Most often, I have patients take magnesium taurate, a form of magnesium that includes the mineral magnesium and taurine. While there is little literature overall, the published articles suggest no toxicity. Since taurine may lower blood pressure and contribute to drowsiness, try taking it at bedtime. Persons taking antihypertension medications should monitor their blood pressure to make sure it doesn't drop too low.

Food Sources of Taurine
Taurine is present only in animal-derived foods. Meats and eggs are top sources.

Theanine

Made from green tea, theanine is known to relax, balance, and really take the pressure off. I mean that literally—theanine is not only calming but also has been shown to lower blood pressure at the same time. It also balances the cortisol-to-DHEA ratio that we measure in saliva tests by lowering cortisol levels when they are too high. Theanine also supports dopamine, GABA, and serotonin activity—three neurotransmitters that can be low with anxiety states. Even more, theanine will generate alpha states, the calming feelings that we attain in meditation and when we are comfortably falling asleep.

Theanine has even been studied when used in conjunction with antipsychotic medications for schizophrenic and schizoaffective patients. Studies found not only no interactions with the medications but also a lowering of the worrisome signs of these conditions, such as delusions, hallucinations, disorganized speech, and paranoia.

Theanine Dosage and Toxicity
Try theanine at 200 mg once or twice a day. This supplement is best for people with obsessive thoughts or anxiety-related high blood pressure. It's great for chronic anxiety, but isn't going to be much help for situational panic attacks. It's been used at 400 mg in boys with ADHD as a sleep aid; try it at this dosage if you're having sleep problems that the other recommendations in this book do not address.

Tryptophan and 5-Hydroxytryptophan (5-HTP)

Rounding out this tour de force of anxiety-helping amino acids are two that are probably the most well known in the natural antianxiety world. Tryptophan and 5-HTP naturally raise serotonin, the neurotransmitter of good mood. Low levels are often present in people with increased panic response, low mood, and depression.

While selective serotonin reuptake inhibitors (SSRIs) can artificially keep levels of serotonin high by poisoning the system that breaks serotonin down, tryptophan and 5-HTP naturally help the body to make more serotonin as needed. This is good for two reasons. One is that the body has more control over the situation, which means fewer side effects. Second, SSRIs are known in the long term to deplete serotonin stores—this is why they often work for a while and then stop working after a year or so. Supplemental 5-HTP and tryptophan do not seem to have this problem.

Despite the widespread use and anecdotal reports from natural doctors like me, there is surprisingly very little research on these amino acids. Much of the research came before the drugs were widely used. I guess once there's a patentable drug compound to make money with, there is less of a motivation to study natural, non-patented versions. That is too bad, for the drugs have clear side effects, and these natural remedies typically do not.

A small double-blind, placebo-controlled, crossover study pilot asked seven social phobia subjects to eat a tryptophan-rich seed for twelve weeks. When these subjects combined the seed with a carbohydrate source, they reported significant anxiety relief. Another double-blind placebo-controlled study from 1987 looked at 5-HTP and the tricyclic antidepressant Anafranil in forty-five anxiety patients. While Anafranil showed superior improvement on all rating scales as compared to a placebo, the 5-HTP held its own, with moderate reduction of symptomatology and best effects on agoraphobia (fear of public places) and panic.

One study of patients using a carbon dioxide inhalation challenge to induce panic in forty-eight subjects (twenty-four panic disorder patients and twenty-four controls) revealed how 200 mg of 5-HTP one and a half hours before the challenge significantly reduced panic reactions, whereas the placebo had no effect. That's impressive. When I was going through my own anxiety and panic issues in my twenties, I tried that carbon dioxide inhalation challenge—basically, it feels as if you are suffocating. Not fun when you are already pretty anxious, I can tell you that.

Tryptophan and 5-HTP Dosage

While tryptophan has been around longer, 5-HTP is considered more potent due to its increased ability to cross the blood-brain barrier. In fact, 5-HTP is about 70 percent absorbed, versus 3 percent for tryptophan, so less 5-HTP is often used. Having said that, I find that some patients see more benefits from tryptophan, while others see more from 5-HTP. So you may need to try them both and see which works better for you. As a general rule, I recommend 5-HTP for daytime anxiety or panic issues, and I dose 100 mg three times a day, away from meals and protein sources, but with a little carbohydrate (like an apple slice or rice cracker) for best absorption into the brain. If 100 mg three times a day doesn't start working for you within two weeks, double the dose to 200 mg three times a day. For trouble sleeping, I dose tryptophan at 1,000 to 2,000 mg at bedtime, especially to help patients *stay* asleep. Tryptophan and 5-HTP also have some great side benefits—they help with depression as well as weight loss, for they seem to moderate the carbohydrate-craving centers of the brain. In comparison, many SSRI drugs do the exact opposite, causing patients to gain weight that is often hard to lose, even after stopping the drug.

Tryptophan and 5-HTP Toxicity

When dosed accordingly, tryptophan appears to be quite safe and effective. Just to let you know, about twenty years ago, there was a lot of misinformation about the safety of tryptophan. In 1989, a few individuals fell ill with eosinophilia myalgia-syndrome (EMS) after consuming the supplement. This syndrome causes of severe muscle and joint pain, high fever, swelling of the arms and legs, weakness, and shortness of breath. Sadly, more than thirty deaths were attributed to EMS caused by tryptophan supplements. Although the supplement itself was originally blamed and then banned in the US, it was actually contaminants that were at fault due to poor quality control—the deaths had nothing to do with the tryptophan, but rather with the company that had no business making supplements. Today, tryptophan is back on the market, and there are absolutely no toxicity issues. Unfortunately, you will still see strong warnings against tryptophan products on the Internet from websites like WebMD. This is likely because big pharma gives huge advertising dollars to WebMD—whenever they can convince you not to use a natural supplement replacement for their drug, they will try to do so—even if they spread misinformation in the process.

More salient to this conversation is the risk of a condition called serotonin syndrome. This is a situation in which SSRIs are used together or in addition to natural therapies, increasing serotonin levels. This syndrome can be characterized by severe agitation, nausea, and confusion and may include hallucinations, increased heart rate, blood pressure changes, feeling hot, coordination issues, hyper reflexes, and/or gastrointestinal tract symptoms like nausea, vomiting, and diarrhea. Severe cases of serotonin syndrome can cause rapid fluctuation of temperature and blood pressure, mental status changes, and even coma.

Again, fears around this syndrome seem to be overblown in regards to supplements. Serotonin syndrome was reported in a study of four elderly patients who supposedly developed the condition as a result of an interaction between the drugs Tramadol and Remeron, two antidepressants. Although polypharmacy (giving too many drugs at the same time) may have caused this syndrome, there have been no reports that natural substances can cause it alone or when used with a conventional medication. With careful dosing of SSRI drugs and tryptophan together, the supplementation may prove a side effect–free integrative approach to anxiety. Of course, I always recommend you let your physician know if you are working with natural supplements and monitor for any serotonin syndrome symptoms. Bring this book to your doctor to show the research that is available about this topic. I have worked with scores of patients using conventional medications with tryptophan and 5-HTP, and I have not seen one issue yet.

Food Sources of Tryptophan and 5-HTP
Tryptophan can be found in small amounts in all foods that contain protein. Relatively high amounts are present in bananas, turkey (which may contribute to the Thanksgiving sleepiness many people experience—although that sleepy effect is more likely due to eating too much food), red meat, dairy, nuts, seeds, soy, tuna, and shellfish. There are no food sources of 5-HTP.

Antianxiety Herbs
Botanical medicines, or herbs, have been used for millennia to treat disease and ease discomfort. Our ancestors learned to use herbal medicines from the animals, who instinctively gravitated toward different plants for different health issues. Today, we have access to thousands of years of anecdotal use of these herbs, combined with powerful research from the last century or so.

While many conventional doctors are scared of herbs, I think herbal medications are fantastic. They are effective and quite safe overall. While conventional medications are easily overdosed, herbal medicines are not as likely to be used in excess, for they have plant chemicals that give gentle signs against overdoing it (like diarrhea or stomach distress). Conventional drugs have no warning signals.

While caution is always prudent, it should also be noted that, according to both research and vast anecdotal usage over thousands of years, herbal medicines seem to have an exemplary safety record. According to Dr. Arthur Presser of the University of Southern California School of Pharmacy, deaths from herbs are extremely rare compared to conventional medicines (or even typical everyday events). He suggests that there are about one in 333 deaths from properly used medications, but only one in one million deaths from the use of herbal remedies.

Number of Deaths per Situation

◆ 1 in 20 deaths from bypass operations

◆ 1 in 250 deaths from medical mishaps

◆ 1 in 333 from properly dosed drugs

◆ 1 in 5,000 deaths from auto accidents

◆ 1 in 1,000,000 deaths from herbal medicines

These numbers are impressive, and underscore the safety of herbs. In today's sound byte world, the media seems to only report on the dangers of these "mysterious plants," but not the relative dullness of herbal safety. For my patients, they are not mysterious—they are cherished friends.

Ashwagandha

We discuss a number of herbs in this book, and ashwagandha (*Withania somnifera*) has the longest and richest history of them all. The word *ashwagandha* translates to "smell of a horse." That clever name points to the herb's historical use of imparting the strength and vitality of our hoofed friends, and it also points to its not-too-pleasant aroma. It is a stinky herb, but it's a good one for anxiety.

Ashwagandha is great for a really stressed-out system. Modern-day research shows ashwagandha's benefits in regards to the nervous system, Parkinson's disease, inflammation, and fertility. Some studies show benefit in helping reverse chemotherapy-induced leucopenia (low white blood cells).

While many animal studies show that ashwagandha can help anxiety, only recently have studies proven its human anxiety-breaking benefits. These studies showed reduced stress scores, cortisol-decreasing effects, and benefits with adrenal hyperplasia (a situation where the adrenal glands have swollen due to chronic stress). Stressed women also found benefit in alopecia (hair loss), while men with fertility concerns enjoyed increased antioxidants and more potent sperm.

Dosage of Ashwagandha

General dosage is 300 mg, standardized up to 5 percent to withanolides (this means that 5 percent of the total amount of the herb you take is made of withanolides, which some researchers think is the active component in this botanical). Having taken ashwagandha myself for a number of months, I noticed that it gave me better quality sleep and made me less reactive to stressful circumstances. While toxicity has not been noted in most studies, there's one case of excess body hair growth that was attributed to the mechanism that raises DHEA levels. I have never seen that effect in the hundreds of women I have worked with who have taken it. I have seen one senior patient vomit from the herb, so some people's digestive tracts may be sensitive to it.

Curcumin

Curcumin, or *Curcuma longa,* is a component of turmeric. This herbal compound enjoys a long and rich history stemming from thousands of years of use in Asian culture. Today, curcumin is hailed for its anticancer properties, nervous system help, and anti-inflammatory benefits. It lowers inflammation in the digestive tract, such as ulcerative colitis, polyp formation, and proctitis. It can even help create new nerve cells in emotional centers of the brain while helping to support antianxiety production of norepinephrine, dopamine, and serotonin. Animal studies show curcumin's significant antianxiety powers in stressed mice, possibly through changes of serotonin expression in the brain.

Curcumin Dosage and Toxicity

If you have anxiety and inflammation (like skin rashes, rheumatoid issues, colitis, or high inflammatory markers such as CRP), curcumin may be a good choice for you. Curcumin extracts that are 90 to 95 percent pure can be taken at 250 mg three times a day. If you suffer from a lot of inflammation, you can double this dosage. While side effects are uncommon, curcumin supplementation may cause mild gastritis or nausea. It is best taken without food.

Kava Kava

Kava (*Piper methysticum*) is widely used in the Western Pacific tradition. Kava translates to "intoxicating pepper." Indeed, it will help calm but will not make a person feel sleepy or foggy in the process. It has an especially profound relaxation effect on the muscles, and as you may know, when muscle tension calms, you feel calmer, too. Also, research suggests that kava can keep dopamine and GABA levels elevated.

Over the last twenty-five years, six quality trials of kava for anxiety patients found anxiety-breaking benefits. These effects were especially strong for women, and the younger a person was, the better it worked. Since the late 1990s, a number of controlled trials have looked at the effectiveness of kava in anxiety.

The Cochrane study group is an independent multinational effort to look objectively at medical research data. The group conducts large studies called meta-analyses that pore through all the available studies on a subject to date to see if they support one another and give a clear picture of what is being studied. One Cochrane meta-analysis looked at eleven kava trials with a total of 645 participants and found kava to be effective versus placebo. Most of the research concluded that when kava is used as an anxiolytic alternative to benzodiazepines or tricyclic antidepressants, individuals typically suffer from fewer side effects. Two studies did not show benefit for kava. Overall, though, the majority of studies show substantial benefit.

Kava has also been researched to help patients safely wean off anti-anxiety medications. A German study utilized a five-week, randomized, placebo-controlled, double-blind study of forty-nine patients given kava for that purpose. During the first treatment week, the kava was increased from 50 mg to 300 mg per day while the patients' benzodiazepine medication was tapered off over two weeks. This was followed by three weeks of 300 mg kava or placebo without medication. Patients were monitored for safety and withdrawal symptoms (dizziness, anxiety, depression, sleeping problems, and so on). The kava was helpful and clearly better than placebo. Also, kava had no side effects.

Kava Kava Dosage and Toxicity

In my office, I usually start with a tincture of kava, giving thirty drops three times a day to help bring relaxation, especially if muscle tension is present. You can place the tincture drops in some water or make a tea with it. As mentioned earlier, kava works better on younger people and women. It is great for muscular tension that often accompanies anxiety. To wean off benzodiazepines with kava, start with 50 mg and move up to 300 mg per day while tapering off the benzodiazepine medication over two weeks. Follow this with three weeks of 300 mg of kava per day.

None of the studies I have talked about found any toxicity, as a review of over 465 studies also concluded. However, in 2002, the FDA had some concern over kava because of a few fatal liver disease cases. Experts in the natural medicine field examined these and believe these were actually not due to kava, but instead to multiple medication use and/or advanced liver disease that was already present in these patients. Given its exceedingly long history of safe use with millions of users in Germany and Switzerland, I also believe it is unlikely that kava was the problem. Nevertheless, to be safe, I recommend that those with liver disease refrain from taking kava, and instead look for another natural relaxant from the choices in this book. If you are concerned, you can have your doctor run liver enzyme tests every month, though I have not seen liver enzymes ever raise with kava supplementation. Interestingly, a few case studies have mentioned that kava increases anxiety. This is known as a paradoxical effect, and I have seen it once or twice in my office as well. This reminds me to honor how each person is unique—what can be good for one person is not always good for someone else.

Lavender

If you have ever smelled lavender, you probably already know that its aroma is relaxing and calming. That is probably the best way to describe it. No wonder it has been such a well-known antianxiety herb for thousands of years! While there's a long usage history, only recently has modern medical science started to look at lavender for anxiety.

One randomized control trial of eighty women who took daily baths with lavender oil experienced improved mood, reduced aggression, and a more positive outlook. A double-blind study compared a lavender gelcap called Silexan to Ativan for generalized anxiety disorder, and reported that about 40 percent of patients who used lavender got better, while only 27 percent who took the Ativan improved—and the lavender had no side effects. Another multicenter study of 221 patients with anxiety also showed clear benefits of an immediate-release capsule preparation of lavender over a placebo. While these studies do seem to hold up on their own merits, several of the authors of both studies were employees of the company making the herbal preparation. Independent studies will need to confirm their findings. I have seen lavender gelcaps work for a majority of patients who take them, but not with everyone.

Lavender Dosage and Toxicity
I recommend the immediate-release gelcaps of 80 mg lavender oil that were used in the studies, or lavender essential oil dropped into a nice Epsom salt bath. Another option is using thirty drops of lavender tincture three times a day in a little water or diluted juice. You can make a delicious calming tea of lavender by steeping one or two teaspoons of herb in a cup or two of water. Lavender tea is great for an upset stomach resulting from nervousness. There is no known toxicity for lavender although some research suggests lavender may have a light estrogen effect on younger boys, so I avoid it in males under age thirteen. When I tried the gelcaps, they gave me a mild and almost pleasant herbal lavender "burp" that a minority of patients who take it will experience.

Mucuna

If you are a jazz music buff, you may know of Mel Tormé, the composer and singer known to his fans as "the velvet fog." Well, mucuna (*Mucuna puriens*) is called "the velvet bean." Macuna is an herb hailing from India and known for its rich history. With over two thousand years of recorded use, modern medicine is just starting to study this herb and use it for mood disorder.

The mucuna bean contains a fair amount of the feel-good neurotransmitter dopamine—more than any other known source. Dopamine is also known as a motivation neurotransmitter. Parkinson's disease patients have low dopamine, and three separate studies recorded positive symptom improvement in patients taking 45 grams of mucuna daily (this equals around 1,500 mg of L-dopamine).

Depressed patients who are also anxious can benefit from extra dopamine, and it appears that supplements containing mucuna may be helpful for these conditions. If you are feeling anxious but at the same time have zero motivation (and/or if you have done well on a drug like Wellbutrin, which raises dopamine preferentially), then mucuna might work for you. Conversely, if you have done well on drugs like Risperdal that block dopamine, then you best stay away from the velvet bean and may do better with lithium, which gently brings dopamine down.

Mucuna Dosage and Toxicity
You can start taking 200 mg daily and move up to 200 mg twice a day after two weeks (this supplies about 120–240 mg of L-dopamine). In my practice, I have found that those patients with panic attacks may also be more likely to have low dopamine, while those with anxiety do not. If you are not sure you have a low dopamine issue, start slowly with this herb—you do not want your symptoms to get worse. In fact, I'd strongly recommend you work with a naturopath or other well-informed herbal practitioner when you take mucuna.

Mucuna may cause bloating or nausea. It should be avoided with anticoagulant (blood thinning) drugs. Also, women with polycystic ovarian syndrome (PCOS) might experience worsening of symptoms due to testosterone boosts from mucuna. There have been reported cases of severe vomiting, palpitations, difficulty falling asleep, delusions, or confusion with mucuna. As I mentioned, to be safe, I would recommend you seek out a knowledgeable practitioner when using this particular botanical medicine.

Passionflower

One of my favorite antianxiety herbs, passionflower (*Passiflora incarnata*) is known around the world for its calming properties. Passionflower is right for you if you experience a constant overthinking and swirling thoughts that turn up the anxiety volume in your brain. Patients who report that their mind is "spinning and reeling" often do well with passionflower. I find that people in their twenties who are anxious because they do not know what to do with their lives do quite well with passionflower—its Latin name means "passion incarnate," and it does seem to help people focus and take control of their lives. I wish I had known about it when I was in my twenties!

Like a natural Xanax, passionflower has alkaloids and flavonoids that affect benzodiazepine receptors in the brain. One 2007 review of 198 people showed that passionflower can have the same effect as benzodiazepine drugs. A double-blind, placebo-controlled study of thirty-six patients compared passionflower with the benzodiazepine

Ativan (Lorazepam) in patients with generalized anxiety disorder. While the pharmaceutical had a quicker onset, both passionflower and Ativan were equally effective. The herb showed fewer side effects. Another study looked at sixty patients given passionflower for anxiety ninety minutes before surgery and found they had much lower anxiety presedation. There were also no negative postoperative side effects or interactions with the anesthesia. Other positive effects were noted in a multicenter, double-blind, placebo-controlled general practice study where 182 patients with anxiety and adjustment disorder were given passionflower along with a few other herbs, including hawthorn (great for the heart) and valerian (great for anxiety-induced sleeping problems).

Passionflower Dosage and Toxicity
Passionflower can be dosed as a tea, in capsules or tablets, or as a liquid tincture. I typically prescribe passionflower in tincture form, using one dropperful (about thirty drops) three times a day, placed in a little water or tea.

Passionflower has no known toxicity when used in common dosages and forms. One study did note minor dizziness, drowsiness, and confusion in a patient. Since it may sedate, I don't recommend combining it with alcohol. Regarding prescription sedatives, it's best to work with a naturopathic physician or other practitioner familiar with combining herbs and drugs. There are no studies of passionflower use in pregnant or lactating women. Also, avoid giving passionflower to children under six months old.

Rhodiola
Like phenibut, rhodiola has a rich history of use in Russia and like ashwagandha, it has a history of supporting a stressed human body. It is adaptogenic, meaning it can lower levels of stress hormones when high or raise them when too low, making it a perfect herb for patients who have dysregulated circadian rhythms. Animal tests of rhodiola show both antianxiety and antidepressant benefits. Interestingly, rhodiola does not seem to act like a natural benzodiazepine, like a number of other supplements discussed in this book. Instead, it seems more of an overall stress system balancer with neuroprotective effects.

University of California researchers gave ten patients with generalized anxiety disorder 340 mg of rhodiola once a day for ten weeks. By the tenth week, anxiety was way down. An Armenian study using 340 mg or more also showed antianxiety benefits. This study found that while all other anxiety parameters increased, self-esteem only improved at 1,340 mg of rhodiola a day. Since self-esteem is worth a lot (if not everything), it is worth increasing the dose above 1,340 mg. For boosting self-esteem, I will often recommend my patients listen to Carolyn Myss's CD set on the subject (see chapter 2) along with rhodiola.

Rhodiola Dosage and Toxicity
Start at 340 mg a day, and if you do not see improvement, move up every two weeks until you reach 1,340 mg. No side effects have been noted at any of the dosages mentioned, even the 1,340 mg dose.

St. John's Wort
Used by Hippocrates for anxiety and depression, St. John's wort is the most studied plant medicine of all time. The Latin name *Hypericum perforatum* means "above a ghost," as this plant was known to ward off evil spirits.

My last book, How Come They're Happy and I'm Not?, goes into depth about St. John's wort's amazing results with depression. It is so useful for depression that even the American Psychiatric Association has acknowledged it "might be considered" as an alternative to pharmaceutical medications—that's pretty much a natural medicine rave from the APA.

While most doctors consider it a "natural SSRI," St. John's wort is really much, much more. Besides acting like a gentle SSRI with fewer side effects, it also protects the nervous system, supports thyroid function, balances blood sugar and neurotransmitter levels, and supports GABA. St. John's wort creates its effect by working in places around the whole body, not just the brain.

While St. John's wort is well studied for depression, newer studies are starting to unearth its antianxiety power. Animal studies in diabetic rats given St. John's wort showed minimized anxiety and depression behaviors. With one study showing anxiety reduction in postmenopausal women, another sixty-person study did not see benefits for obsessive-compulsive disorder.

St. John's Wort Dosage and Toxicity

St. John's wort is usually dosed in capsules that range between 900 mg and 1,800 mg of standardized extract, divided into two or three doses per day. Look for a preparation standardized to 0.3 percent of the compound hypericin. Its best use is for people who have "anxious depression"—a combination of depression and strong anxiety. It is not clear to me whether anxiety by itself will benefit, but it may be worth a try if other options do not work for you.

While quite safe from a side effect standpoint, the only concern about St. John's wort is that it can dramatically change the effect of other medications—for good *and* bad. Two studies show how it can help Plavix, an anticlotting drug, work better—in some patients St. John's wort actually helped low doses of Plavix work, preventing them from having to move to doses that could cause side effects.

More concerning is that there is a laundry list of drugs St. John's wort may interact with in a negative way. It has been known to conflict with the effectiveness of birth control—in fact, unbeknownst to me, my sister-in-law was taking St. John's wort while on birth control pills. She became pregnant, and I have two wonderful twin nephews as a result. Even though, in the end, it was a happy interaction for our family, it does underscore the need to talk to your doctor or pharmacist before starting St. John's wort if you are taking other medications. Photosensitivity has occurred in some HIV patients on antiviral drugs as well.

Summary Charts of Supplements for Easy Reference

General Supplementation for All Patients

Supplement	Best use	Typical dosage	Possible side effects	Toxicity, contraindication, interactions	Food sources
Multiple vitamin	General anxiety	Follow dosage on bottle	None known	None known	Vegetables and fruits
Fish oil	Anxiety; high CRP	About 2 grams 1x/day; ~1,000 mg a day of EPA and about 800 mg of DHA	Possible reflux	No known toxicity; contraindicated if allergic to fish or if taking anticlotting medications	Fish
Probiotics	General anxiety and depression support	Lactobacillus acidophilus and bifidobacter lactis capsules of 4–8 billion living organisms, 1–3x/day	None known	None known	Natto, kim chi, miso, sauerkraut

Vitamin Supplementation

Supplement	Best use	Typical dosage	Possible side effects	Toxicity, contraindication, interactions	Food sources
Vitamin B3 (niacinamide form)	Panic, anxiety, and OCD; benefits for staying asleep when used with tryptophan	100 mg 3x/ day	None known	Long-term use should include precautionary monitoring of liver enzymes; use may increase effectiveness of tryptophan; avoid with anticonvulsant medications	Chicken, turkey, beef, liver, peanuts, sunflower seeds, mushrooms, avocado, green peas
Vitamin B6 (pyridoxine)	Anxiety and depression	25 mg to 50 mg 1x/day; may work best when taken with magnesium	200 mg or more a day may cause a reversible hand and food tingling and/or fatigue	Birth control pills can lower B6 levels	Bell peppers, spinach, potatoes, bananas, turnip greens
Vitamin B12 (methylcobalamin)	Anxiety and depression; support for treatment-resistant depression	1 mg 1x/day	Will occasionally cause insomnia if taken too late in the day	Metformin can lower B12 status	Snapper, calf's liver, venison, shrimp, scallops, salmon, beef
Folic acid (methylfolate)	Depression and reatment-resistant depression	400–1,000 mcg or 5–15 mg 1x/day for treatment-resistant depression	None known	Avoid when taking methotrexate for cancer treatment; avoid with epilepsy medications; can help antidepressants work better	Spinach, asparagus, romaine lettuce, turnip greens, mustard greens, calf's liver, collard greens, cauliflower, broccoli, parsley, lentils, beets

Inositol	May be best for panic disorder	6–18 grams 1x/day	Minor gastric discomfort	None known	Most vegetables, nuts, wheat germ, brewers yeast, bananas, liver, brown rice, oat flakes, unrefined molasses, raisins
B complex	General daily stress support for nonanxious people; supports depression and anxiety; high homocysteine	40 mg of vitamin B6, 1.2 mg of B12 in the methylcobalamin form, and folate (in the form of l-methyltetrahydrofolate) at 2 grams per day	High levels of B6 can cause reversible neuropathy symptoms	None known	Vegetables, whole grains, beans

Mineral Supplementation

Supplement	Best use	Typical dosage	Possible side effects	Toxicity, contraindication, interactions	Food sources
Magnesium glycinate	Sleep issues; anxiety	250 mg 2x/day	Possible loose stools if sensitive	None known	None
Magnesium taurate	Depression; anxiety	300–700 mg; or one to two cups in a warm bath	Can cause loose stools in sensitive individuals	Kidney disease; diarrhea	None
Chromium	Anxiety and/or depression that correlates with hypo- or hyperglycemia	200–600 mcg/day total, taken in divided doses with meals	None known at recommended dosages	Monitor for lowering of blood sugar in patients using diabetic medications	None
Selenium	Anxiety and/or depression with low thyroid function or low T3	100–200 mcg 1x/day	Doses larger than 400 mcg may cause symptoms of dermatitis, hair loss, and brittle nails	None known	Tuna, meat, fish, nuts (especially Brazil nuts), garlic
Lithium orotate	Anxiety or depression, especially in patients who benefit from oxytocin-related treatments like massage	5–20 mg of elemental lithium per day	Common supplemental doses show no toxicity; high doses can cause muscle weakness, loss of appetite, mild apathy, tremors, nausea, and vomiting	Impaired kidney function	None

put anxiety behind you

| Zinc | Treatment-resistant depression; leaky gut; supports the immune system and skin | 15 mg 2x/day—use zinc carnosine form for leaky gut | Can cause nausea when taken on an empty stomach or in sensitive individuals | Large doses (greater than 150 mg a day) can cause vomiting and loss of appetite; long-term consumption may deplete copper. Balance with 2 mg of copper 1x/day if taking for more than two months. Do not add copper if blood copper levels are high | None |

Amino Acid Supplementation

Supplement	Best use	Typical dosage	Possible side effects	Toxicity, contraindication, interactions	Food sources
L-Carnitine or acetyl-L-carnitine	Depression and/or anxiety; provides cognitive support in seniors; works for postpartum anxiety	L-carnitine form 500–1,500 mg 2x/day to raise serum carnitine; acetyl-L-carnitine at 1 to 3 grams for raising serum carnitine and for cognitive support	None known	Can help prevent deficiency from anticonvulsant medications	Predominantly animal sources: beef, chicken, turkey, pork, lamb, fish
Gamma amino-butyric acid (GABA)	Anxiety, insomnia	100–200 mg up to 3x/day, away from food; take no more than 1,000 mg within a four-hour period and no more than 3,000 mg within a twenty-four-hour period	Dizziness and sleepiness	Rare: bruising and bleeding at high doses	Green, black, and oolong teas, fermented foods like yogurt, oats, whole grains, brown rice
Phenibut	Anxiety, insomnia	300–900 mg 1x/day for anxiety or for anticipated stress	Dizziness and sleepiness	Avoid taking long term (need breaks every two weeks); can be addictive	None
Glycine	Anxiety; anticipated panic situations	5–10 grams (one to two teaspoons) 1x/day or before a stressful situation; can be mixed with passionflower	None known	Check with a doctor before using if liver or kidney disease is present; may be beneficial for schizophrenia	Fish, meat, beans, dairy

put anxiety behind you

Supplement	Condition	Dosage	Side effects	Notes	Food sources
Lysine and arginine	Anxiety in stress situations	2 to 3 grams of each 2x/day, away from food	High doses (20–30 grams) of arginine may cause diarrhea	Arginine may be contraindicated with type I herpetic sores or heart attack history	Nuts, red meat, spinach, lentils, whole grains, chocolate, eggs, seafood, soy
N-acetyl-cysteine (NAC)	Obsessive compulsive disorder, gambling issues, and trichotillomania (hair pulling); may benefit bipolar disorder; helps with sinus congestion, too	500–600 mg 2–3x/day	Occasional headache or stomach discomfort	Helps as an adjunct to risperidone for irritability symptoms	Cysteine precursor found in high-protein foods (meats, tofu, eggs, dairy products)
Phosphatidylserine	Anxiety and depression; chronically high or low cortisol; chronic high stress	200–800 mg a day in divided doses on an empty stomach; combines well with essential fatty acids	None known	May benefit high liver enzymes	Organ meats (liver and kidney), mackerel, herring, tuna, soft-shell clams, white beans
Taurine	Anxiety with low energy and cardiovascular concerns	500 mg up to 3x/day or in the form of magnesium taurate	Headaches, nausea, nosebleeds, temporary balance disturbance	Possible blood pressure-lowering effects; monitor when taking blood pressure medications	Meat and eggs
L-theanine	Anxiety with chronic running or obsessive thoughts	200–400 mg 1x/day, away from food	None known	May increase effects of some chemotherapy	Green tea

Tryptophan	Trouble staying asleep	500–2,500 mg 1x/day, take away from food, but with a high-glycemic simple carbohydrate	Morning drowsiness	None known, when used with Prozac one study showed benefit without interaction; monitor for serotonin syndrome when used with SSRIs and tricyclics	Small amounts in pumpkin seeds, bananas, turkey
5-HTP	Anxiety, especially agoraphobia and panic; depression with a social anxiety or panic component	100–200 mg 3x/day, taken on an empty stomach; take 200 mg of 5-HTP 1.5 hours before anticipated panic attack	Nausea and occasional vomiting	May increase diarrhea symptoms; monitor for serotonin syndrome when used with SSRIs and tricyclics	None

Herbal Remedies

Supplement	Best use	Typical dosage	Possible side effects	Toxicity, contraindication, interactions	Food sources
Ashwagandha	Chronic anxiety; alopecia; low sperm count	300 mg (withanolide content of at least 1 to 5 percent) 1–2x/day	Vomiting and gastric distress in some patients	Watch for excessive hair growth and increased DHEA levels in women	None
Curcumin	Inflammation; leaky gut; depression; possible anxiety benefit	1,000 mg 1x/day of the BCM-95 form, away from meals	Nausea and gastritis are rare	None known; studied for its benefits adjunctively with fluoxetine and imipramine	Turmeric spice
Kava kava	Anxiety, especially with muscle tension and in women with interstitial cystitis; for weaning off benzodiazepine medications	Tincture dose of 30 drops 2–3x/day in water or as a tea; 400 mg 1x/day extract	Paradoxical increase in anxiety symptoms in small percentage of users	Should be avoided in patients with liver disease	None
Lavender	Anxiety, especially with a "nervous stomach"	80 mg immediate release oil; one or two teaspoons per cup of tea; 30 drops of tincture 3x/day; essential oil on the pillow at night or in a warm bath	May cause mild "lavender burp"	Studied for benefit when used with SSRI and tricylic medications for depression	None

Macuna	Depression with anxiety, especially in patients who do well with dopamine-boosting drugs Some patients with panic attacks may also benefit	200 mg of the extract; after two weeks, up to 200 mg 2x/day	Bloating and nausea; high doses can cause vomiting, palpitations, difficulty sleeping, delusions, or confusion	Best used with professional supervision. Avoid with Parkinson's medications, anticoagulant medications; contraindicated in PCOS; consult with practitioner if taking antidepressant medications	None
Passionflower	Anxiety; generalized anxiety disorder	1 dropperful of tincture (about 30 drops) 3x/day	Unlikely, but possible minor dizziness, drowsiness, and confusion	Do not combine with alcohol; if using sedatives, work with a practitioner; avoid with MAO-inhibiting antidepressant drugs	None
Rhodiola	Anxiety; generalized anxiety and depression; helpful for feelings of burnout and self-esteem challenges	340–1,340 mg 1x/day, standardized for 1 percent of rosavin	Possible dry mouth and dizziness	None known	None
St. John's wort	Depression; depression with anxiety; postmenopausal depression; may help lower blood sugar levels in diabetics	900–1,800 mg of standardized extract per day	Photosensitivity	Can enhance or reduce effectiveness of many drugs that are affected by the P450 system; improves effectiveness of clopidogrel (Plavix)	None

Antianxiety Homeopathics

The term "homeopathy" is derived from the Greek words *homeo*, which means similar, and *pathos*, which means suffering. Homeopathy is considered a cheap, safe way to effect great changes in a person's underlying energetic patterns to bring healing. For those who distrust "alternative medicine," homeopathy is usually the natural medicine brought under the most scrutiny, for, admittedly, it is hard to believe and easy to discredit.

Whether you believe in it or not, homeopathic treatments have remained a part of successful care in Europe and India for over one hundred years. Homeopathy was developed by Samuel Hahnemann, a medical doctor, in the late eighteenth century. Interestingly, Hahnemann is the namesake of Hahnemann Medical School in Pennsylvania, where homeopathy has not been taught since the 1920s, when the American Medical Association ran natural medicine out of town, and eventually out of the country. That's another interesting story— if you want to know more, check out my blog post, "The Flexner Report: How It Affects Your Healthcare Today," on my Psychology Today blog at *www.psychologytoday.com.*

Homeopathy is a system of remedies that will help bring physiologic change to the body when used in minute, or even infinitesimally diluted doses. Despite the American Medical Association's wish to squash anything related to natural medicine, by the second half of the nineteenth century, homeopathy continued to grow and gain acceptance. With a reputation for efficacy, it spread throughout Europe, Asia, and North America. Today, it is well accepted in India and Germany for use along with conventional care.

The studies of homeopathic medicines for mood are limited. Probably one of the strongest studies to date for homeopathic treatment of anxiety and depression is a 1997 study out of Duke university that looked at remedies given to twelve adults who had major depression, social phobia, or panic disorder. The outpatient subjects either requested homeopathic treatment or received it on a physician's recommendation after partial or poor response to conventional therapies.

Patients were prescribed individual homeopathic prescriptions based on their presentations. Treatment ranged from seven to eight weeks. Overall response rates were 58 percent for overall improvement and 50 percent for phobia ratings. Because it was an uncontrolled trial, it's difficult to truly know how well it worked. The authors concluded that homeopathy "may be useful in the treatment of affective and anxiety disorders in patients with mildly to severely symptomatic conditions." While not definitive, it was deemed valuable by a 2005 independent study review.

One 2013 randomized, double-blind, placebo-controlled study looked at a combination of homeopathic remedies for stressed women. For fourteen days, forty female subjects took three tablets of a homeopathic that included respinum, gelsemium, passiflora, coffea, and veratrum. On the fifteenth day of the study, participants took three pills in the morning and upon arrival at the study site. Patients were assessed for salivary cortisol, plasma cortisol, and epinephrine and heart rates, as well as anxiety, stress, and insecurity. While cortisol levels did not differ between groups, homeopathically treated participants enjoyed better sleep quality and lower epinephrine levels. The authors concluded that the homeopathic helped regulate the neuroendocrine stress response during acute stress and impaired sleep.

A meta-analysis on homeopathy was conducted by Duke's Wayne Jonas, former head of the Office of Alternative Medicine at NIH and a conventional physician who also uses natural medicines and homeopathy. Jonas and his team looked at twenty-five homeopathic studies with over 1,431 volunteers who took homeopathic remedies. They found benefit for physical ailments like fibromyalgia and chronic fatigue syndrome, but there didn't seem to be much positive help for anxiety and stress. Looking at other psychiatric disorders, homeopathy produced mixed effects.

As we can see, when studying homeopathy using conventional parameters you get a mixed bag, with some suggestion of efficacy. It is highly possible that studying homeopathy using a more holistic, systems-based paradigm might show better results. For now, it is unclear whether homeopathy may work for you. My clinical experience tells me it is quite safe and certainly worth trying.

Dosage of Homeopathics

One simple, low-potency approach to dosing homeopathics is to take one dose of 30X or 30C (where X is a dilution of 10 and C is a dilution of 100) potency every six to twelve hours. Look for change in your symptoms over the next week, and stop taking the remedy once symptoms are better. If there is no change in your symptoms, consider choosing another remedy. If symptoms worsen with any dose, no matter how light, then you should consider another remedy.

Below, I have listed the top homeopathic anxiety remedies I use. Scan these to see if any of them fit your profile. Probably not every single element of a description will fit, but you may resonate with one overall pattern. If you are interested in homeopathy, you may want to purchase a homeopathic *materia medica,* which breaks down the remedies into greater detail. Also consider working with a certified homeopath. Please see appendix II for resources to find one.

Aconite Napellus
+ Symptoms of panic and anxiety come on suddenly
+ High temperature/fever
+ Feeling like you are going to die
+ Pounding heart
+ Shock that gets to your core

Argentum Nitricum
+ Generalized anxiety disorder
+ Chronic anxiety
+ Dizziness
+ Chronic worrying
+ Fear of heights
+ Heart palpitations

Arsenicum Album
+ Anxiety about safety
+ Concerned with being robbed or financial security
+ Type A personality—impatient, interrupts others, walks and talks at a fast pace
+ Perfectionist, has expectations for self and others that are typically not met
+ Demanding
+ Curt or rude

- Enjoys company
- Feels better in warm weather
- Shortness of breath

Calcarea Carbonica

- Fear of changes
- Feeling overwhelmed by physical illness
- Afraid of losing control
- Afraid of animals and insects
- Perspires easily, especially while eating and working
- Feels chilly and sluggish and easily tired with exertion
- Open air and the outdoors make you feel better, while stuffy rooms will make symptoms worse
- Craves rich and fatty foods; eggs

Coffea Cruda

- Anxiety with insomnia
- Restlessness, nervous agitation
- Racing mind
- Does poorly with surprise
- Does poorly with pain
- Tends to have nerve pain
- Feels better when lying down
- Worse pain or anxiety with night, odors, noise

Gelsemium

- Agoraphobia
- Muscular weakness from performance anxiety
- Overall fatigue
- Muscular shakiness and trembling
- Hot flashes

Ignatia
+ Anxiety with mood swings
+ Anxiety with menopause
+ Feelings of a lump in the throat and heaviness in the chest
+ Insomnia (or excessive sleeping), headaches, and cramping pains in the abdomen and back
+ Frequently sighing or yawning

Kali Arsenicosum
+ Anxiety, especially about cardiovascular problems
+ Worse symptoms at night; will avoid bed
+ Often feels cold
+ Might sleep holding hand over the heart area

Kali Phosphoricum
+ Anxiety with a sense of being overwhelmed
+ Easy to startle or frighten
+ Great sensitivity
+ Irritable or exhausted from anxiety
+ Fears of having a nervous breakdown
+ Fears that something bad is going to happen

Lycopodium
+ Low self-esteem and confidence
+ Anxiety with being in front of an audience
+ Little self-confidence and may talk too much to compensate
+ Loves sweets
+ Flatulence and stomach upset
+ Bed-wetting in children

Natrum Muriaticum
+ Reserved and quiet, with anxiety
+ Isolated
+ Anxiety with chest pains

- Easily hurt
- Holds grudge
- Refuses help, but is sympathetic to others
- Migraines
- Insomnia

Phosphorus
- Greatest fear is being alone with anxiety compounded by loneliness
- Loves company
- Highly social and likeable
- Highly imaginative
- Affected by odors and noise
- Prefers cold

Pulsatilla
- Childlike sweetness
- Clingy and teary anxiousness
- Loves to be consoled
- Painful premenstrual symptoms and menses
- Thick mucus discharge (nasal, vaginal)

Silica
- Oversensitivity brings on sense of dread
- New task or situation can bring anxiety easily
- Thin frame and osteoporosis
- Frailty
- Responsible and diligent
- Low stamina and easily sickened from overwork

Veratrum
- Low mood with anxiety (anxious depression)
- Feels a sense of collapse
- Feels a sense of coldness

- ◆ May have strong vomiting
- ◆ Perspires easily when uncomfortable
- ◆ Bothered by wet or cold weather
- ◆ Often hungry

Strategy to Discontinue Medications

As with any addictive medicine, antianxiety medications are tough to stop once you start taking them. Our brains and bodies become dependent on them, and withdrawing from them without a negative experience is nearly impossible. The experience of "discontinuation syndrome" (the medical term for what really is withdrawal) is a major challenge for both antidepressant and antianxiety medications. Symptoms include depression, anxiety, confusion, irritability, dizziness, lack of coordination, sleeping problems, crying spells, and blurry vision.

If you have thought about or even tried getting off medications, but did not succeed due to side effects or a return of the original symptoms, do not fear—I have a plan for you.

Step 1: Don't Change a Thing

I know this sounds counterintuitive, but hear me out. I am so glad you are reading this book. And while I have successfully helped many people with their anxiety, the truth is that I do not know your particular situation or personal story. But if you were my family member, friend, or patient, I would tell you the same thing: it is important that your prescribing doctor knows you are ready to try life without antianxiety medication. As such, I want you to work with someone who knows your personal story, and who can make sure your symptoms are stable and guide you as you wean off medications. Do not do this on your own—some people with severe anxiety need to stay on medications longer than they think is necessary. And some patients who have complicating psychiatric issues like schizophrenia or bipolar should not stop taking medications without thoughtful consideration of the benefits and drawbacks of such a change. So please, check with your prescribing doctor to make sure you are ready.

When we get to this conversation, some of my patients will say to me, "but I can't talk to my doctor." If you do not feel that you have a good relationship with your prescribing doctor, then **start looking**

for another doctor you feel you can talk to. Remember, your health is on the line and you deserve someone in your corner whom you trust. There are many gentle, caring psychiatrists and conventional docs out there. You many need to interview a few, but you will find the one who is right for you.

Step 2: Follow the Naturopathic Path

This book covers diet, lifestyle, stress, sleep, nutrients, botanicals, and much more. If you do not read about these things and try to integrate them into your life as best you can, you cannot expect your body to be able to wean off medications. As a general rule, you should follow your naturopathic regimen for at least four months. Generally, I find that after a few months, my patients who are still on medications start to talk me about the idea of discontinuing them. That indicates to me that they have experienced a mental and physical shift, and we can get started on the road to safely weaning off the medications. This shift is not always tangible, but when it happens, you will know it. I usually recommend that once you have added the recommendations and feel that shift, you wait at least another month or two to make sure that it's for real.

Step 3: Supplements to Support the Weaning Process

This is the step where we add a few things to help your body get up to neurotransmitter speed. The general idea is to gently support your body by giving it amino acids and herbal treatments to allow for the eventual transition back to its own mood balance.

The chart below lists medications next to the corresponding related amino acids that help your body create its own neurotransmitters. These amino acids and herbs are putting out little steps for your nervous and hormonal systems to brace themselves as they move down the path to a medication-free life.

If you are ready to wean off:	Use these for at least two months, while slowly tapering off your medication with your doctor's help:
SSRIs: Citalopram (Celexa), Escitalopram (Lexapro), Fluoxetine (Prozac, Prozac Weekly, Sarafem), Paroxetine (Paxil, Paxil CR, Pexeva), Sertraline (Zoloft) Azapirones: Buspirone (Buspar)	1. One month prior to tapering off your prescription medication, start taking 50 mg of 5-HTP and 300 mg of St. John's wort 1x/day for one week. (Remember to check with your doctor before combining St. John's wort with other medications.) Then increase the dose to 2x/day for three weeks. 2. Now slowly start to wean off medication with your prescribing doctor's support. This weaning process should take a minimum of 8 to 12 weeks and the rate will depend on the medication you are taking and the dosage at which you are starting. I generally recommend going twice as slow as prescribed. 3. If you experience withdrawal symptoms like headaches, "zapping" sensations, nausea, sleeping problems, or anxiety, add a third dose of 50 mg 5-HTP with another 300 mg St. John's wort 1x/day. If the symptoms do not get better, you may need to increase the medication up one dose for a week or two until symptoms subside, then continue onward. 4. Once the medication is completed, continue with the supplements for at least one month at the current dose. Then once a week, remove a capsule of either 5-HTP or St. John's wort. After 4 to 6 weeks, you should have completed your weaning process. If some symptoms return while weaning off the supplements, increase the dose back up and remain for two weeks symptom-free, then continue back down in this slow fashion.

| Benzodiazepines: Lorazepam (Ativan), Alprazolam (Xanax), Clonazepam (Klonopin), Clorazepate (Tranxene), Chlordiazepoxide (Librium), Diazepam (Valium), Oxazepam (Serax), Temazepam (Restoril) | **Kava**
Start with 50 mg and move up to 300 mg 1x/day while tapering off the benzodiazepines over two weeks, with a subsequent three weeks of 300 mg of kava 1x/day.

Valerian
For sleeping concern, take 100 mg 3x/day for two weeks before starting to wean off benzodiazepines. Once weaning is complete, stay on valerian for two more weeks, then reduce to 1 capsule a day for one more week. |

8

challenge the anxiety

Making friends with our own demons and their accompanying
insecurity leads to a very simple, understated relaxation and joy.
—Pema Chödrön

Case: Sean

Sean visited me for the first time at age thirty-one with
both generalized anxiety and a fear of traveling away from his
hometown in Long Island, New York. Given the clear, long-
standing digestive issues linked to his anxious feeling, we ran
some digestive tests and found Sean had leaky gut. Using the
protocol of herbs, food, and meditation we talked about in
chapter 5, Sean was able to greatly improve his anxiety levels
in about eight weeks. He felt calmer, but he was still stuck. It
seems with this history of anxiety, he became sensitized to leaving places familiar to him, and even though I thought he was
better, he couldn't shake the fear response that had become
such a habit. It wrecked his social life, and he was always worried that if he lost his job, which was near his house, he would
not be able to go anywhere else to work.

Sean and I mapped out an anxiety strategy. Sean thought about all the possible routes out of town—by means of walking, biking, or driving—and how he would traverse these with his family members and by himself. We rated each scenario on a scale of 1 to 10, with 10 being the most anxiety-provoking. Once armed with this list, Sean started to try the routes one at a time, making sure he moved through each, and not leaving the situation until the anxiety subsided. Sean found taking a teaspoon of glycine and a little passionflower tincture a half hour before his outing was helpful to take the edge off. Sean worked hard on this. Today, Sean is okay to go anywhere he likes. What this teaches us is that for some people, even when the physical issues that originally caused the anxiety improve, the pattern of anxiety may continue. I am proud of Sean, and all my patients, as we learn together how to muster courage to face the anxiety head-on and change those anxious thoughts.

Steps to Overcome Your Anxiety

In chapter 2, we talked about the importance of bringing in new ideas, identifying negative messages, changing those messages, and "thinking like a Buddhist" in order to reframe your anxious thoughts. Chapters 3 through 7 detailed what you need to optimize your physical and overall health: sleep, exercise, nutrients, digestion, blood sugar, mind-body work, and supplements. Now that you have done all this, you can feel confident that your well-supported body is going to allow you to face your fears and anxiety and move through in the best way possible. If you have general anxiety issues, then this chapter may not be necessary for you. You may simply need to work on all the things we have already discussed and give them time to fully take hold and bring your anxiety to zero. But if you have situational anxiety, anxiety about being alone, agoraphobia, or panic issues, this chapter is mandatory reading.

This modern world has a general approach to anxiety and fear: ignore it, avoid it, or take a drug to not feel it. These methods actually keep fear, anxiety, and panic going. These methods send ourselves the message that the fear is too great to handle, and avoidance is the only thing that will help us feel better. This only fortifies the anxiety and robs us of our life.

In Pema Chödrön's book, *When Things Fall Apart,* she tells us that "the most heartbreaking thing of all is how we cheat ourselves of the present moment." Chödrön reminds us that the bravest and most courageous people are not without fear, but instead move toward painful situations, consciously *feeling* the fear they have been avoiding. When people move toward the fear, they do it with compassion for themselves.

You have what it takes—you can be the bravest, too. This is where you are going . . . you are going to feel the fear, have compassion and love for yourself in that present moment, and go ahead with the things you want to do anyway. Once you are done, you will feel exhilarated and in touch with the world.

Step 1: Make a List of What Makes You Fearful

If driving is the issue, you may need to create a list of all the different driving scenarios that are problematic for you. This may include driving on scary routes, being a passenger, or just being near a car. Make the list and rate the items on a scale of 1 to 100. A 100 means it is the most scary, and 1 is the least. For example:

Driving on a service road—65

Driving on the street in front of my house—25

Sitting in the car while it's running—10

Driving over large bridges—100

Sitting in the passenger seat on the highway—40

Driving on the highway—85

Driving on my town's main street—45

Organize the items from the least anxiety-provoking to the most:

Sitting in the car while it's running—10

Driving on the street in front of my house—25

Sitting in the passenger seat on the highway—40

Driving on my town's main street—45

Driving on a service road—65

Driving on the highway—85

Driving over large bridges—100

Let's say you experience agoraphobia. Think about the situations that might cause anxiety for you. This is a real list from a patient of mine:

Swimming in the backyard pool with a loved one—8

Going to the supermarket with a loved one—20

Running outside and feeling my heart beat hard—25

Going to the therapist by myself—35

Going to the supermarket by myself—40

Being home alone during the day—60

Swimming in the pool alone—70

Driving my daughter to school—75

Being home alone at night—95

Step 2: Experience Your Fears, One at a Time

> There's no such thing as insignificant improvement.
> —Tom Peters

Now you can begin your journey to face the fear. This is the journey back to who you are. Instead of running from the fear, you are going to stay with it. As you do, I want you to have total compassion and love for yourself. Most of the time, when we experience anxiety, we hate ourselves and feel ashamed. This time, use the feeling of fear to remind yourself of the love and acceptance you have for yourself. This fear is going to be the foundation of your new courage.

There's a great book called *Feel the Fear and Do It Anyway* by Susan Jeffers. The title gets at the main idea—to know that you can and will feel that fear and that it will not stop you. One of the greatest sporting moments of all time came when Muhammad Ali fought the great George Foreman (yes, of the famous George Foreman Grill), who was holding the heavyweight title Ali wanted so badly. At that point in his career, everyone thought Ali was washed up, and Foreman looked unbeatable. Ali took grueling punches for a few rounds, and at one point looked stuck on the ropes as Foreman pummeled him. Even Ali's own corner thought he was finished. Foreman knew he had Ali—it was just a matter of when. Suddenly, in the midst of

Foreman's salvo in round seven, Ali poked his head up and said to Foreman, "George, that's all you got? I thought you was bad. Show me something. Hit me harder."

Ali ended up demoralizing poor Foreman, who realized that he had already given Ali all he had, and there was no way Ali was going down. Ali stunned Foreman with a combination and Foreman ended up hitting the canvas hard after a few more Ali right hands.

By pretending he was down to lull his opponent into a false sense of security, Ali used what would be known as the "rope-a-dope" fighting style to beat his opponent. You, too, are going to go out, face your fear, take a few punches, and ask your anxiety: "Anxiety, is that all you got? I thought you was bad. Show me something, and hit me harder."

As you say those words, feel free to speak to your anxiety out loud. You know that anxiety has hit you as hard as it can, and you are still here—and only getting better.

To rope-a-dope anxiety out of your life, pick the easiest item first and set a schedule to start working on it. For a person with a fear of driving, this may be sitting in the car while it is running and just getting used to it. If you haven't driven for a long time, even putting the key in the door might be really scary. For an agoraphobic, a good start might be just getting into the backyard pool with someone around or taking a walk down the block and back. Some people who have social anxiety may feel better doing things alone first. For me, driving with someone in the car was more anxiety-provoking than being alone. We are all different, which is why we must create our own anxiety-breaking task list.

Remember to always pick something that is a bit scary for you but not over-the-top scary. When you challenge your George Foreman–sized anxiety, it is critical to feel that fear, know that your mind is creating it, and it cannot really hurt you. And remember that no matter what happens, it will pass. Do not leave the situation until you feel it calm down first. Leaving early will only teach your body that that scary thing really needed to be avoided—this will reinforce the anxiety. If you let it move through and calm, you will learn the situation is under control. And always remember, going out and trying is what is important—*every* outing is a success—no matter the result. In time, you can succeed.

If you are not quite convinced you are ready to challenge yourself, read the next step to help support the process a little bit more.

Step 3: Add a Fear-Supporting Supplement

For many of my patients, I also recommend they increase their anxiety-busting supplements when they start work on their lists. My favorite is the simple combination of a teaspoon (5 grams) of glycine with thirty drops of passionflower in a little water. You can take it about a half hour before going out to face and feel the fear. It will help you adjust to the fear—you will feel it and move through it easier. For those with very strong anxiety, I also recommend 300–600 mg of phenibut a half hour before moving on to the anxious moment. This will help "take the edge off" the event and allow you to work through it a bit easier, without suppressing your feelings or journey through it.

As we have noted, doctors often prescribe antianxiety medications like Xanax and Ativan as a way to suppress the stress response. This is not what we are doing here. The natural supplements are gentle, and in my experience with patients, they do not suppress emotion. Supplements help bring the anxiety down a few notches and allow you to experience that compassionate fear experience that allows you to get to know your bravest self. Eventually, you will be able to face the fear without the supplements. That will be a good feeling.

Summary Checklist

While you move through your list, check in on your thoughts. Be supported by your sleep, foods, exercise, supplements, and mind-body work. You are going at anxiety not from one perspective but from many.

The following is a summary checklist for you to use as you face your fear. Please remember that each number is a pillar for lowering anxiety. Do not skip any of these—they work synergistically to lower anxiety.

1. My new thoughts book (use the list from chapter 2)
2. My sleep schedule
3. My exercise schedule

4. My small, frequent meal schedule

   Breakfast:

   Snack:

   Lunch:

   Snack:

   Dinner:

   Snack:

   Healthy foods I am focusing on:

   Foods I am minimizing:

5. My meditation schedule

6. My mind-body work

7. My basic supplementation

   Multiple vitamin

   Fish oil

   Probiotic

8. My specific anxiety supplements

   Choose which supplements are right for my particular needs

9. My courageous fear-facing plan

   Make a list of what makes me fearful

   Experience fear one step at a time

   Add a supplement for calming, if needed

checking under the hood: lab tests

When a car is making a knocking sound, you don't just look at the car, you open up the hood and see what's going on in there. Anxiety and mood issues are the same. While lab testing by itself doesn't give the whole picture, it can really help us figure out where some of the anxiety is coming from.

In chapter 1, I recommended a few blood tests. The complete list is below. Please note that your doctor may not be able to run all of the tests; sometimes he or she cannot do so for insurance reasons or because the tests are outside of his or her area of expertise. It may be helpful to bring your doctor a copy of this book to help him or her understand the reason you are asking for the test and how to help guide you when the results come back.

Just try to get as many of the blood tests on this list as you can. Remember, there is no one blood test that will make or break your condition, so it is okay if you cannot get them all.

Also, this appendix contains some heavy-duty medical mumbo jumbo. If you don't feel like wading through it, that is fine—just take the below list to your naturopath or other holistic doctor and let them worry about the explanations. If any of your results are not in the normal range, your doctor can explain what to do, and the information below can help guide you when needed.

Blood Work List

Blood sugar panel:

    Fasting blood sugar
    HgBA1C
    Serum insulin

CBC and comp metabolic panel

Cholesterol panel

ABO blood type and Rh test

Inflammation panel:

    Homocysteine
    CRP
    Whole blood histamine

Iron panel:

    Ferritin
    TIBC
    Transferrin
    Serum iron

Hormonal panel:

    TSH
    Free and total T3, T4
    Reverse T3
    Anti-TPO antibodies
    Anti-thyroglobulin antibodies
    PTH
    Serum cortisol
    DHEA
    DHEAs
    Testosterone: free and total
    Serum estrogen and progesterone

Celiac panel:

    Antigliadin antibodies IgG
    Antigliadin antibodies IgM
    TTG
    Secretory IgA

Nutrient panel:

    Serum carnitine
    Serum folic acid
    Serum B12
    Serum 25 (OH) vitamin D
    Plasma zinc
    Serum copper

Genetic testing:

    COMT (catechol-O-methyltransferase)
      Genetic SNP test
    MTHFR gene test

Salivary adrendal panel

Urine kryptopyrroles

Blood toxicity panel:

    GGT
      Serum mercury
      Serum lead
      Serum cadmium
      Serum aluminum

Other toxicity testing:

    Hair analysis and urine testing

    Mold analysis testing

Blood Sugar Panel: Fasting Blood Sugar, Hemoglobin A1C, and Serum Insulin

One of the first tests I recommend is the fasting blood sugar check. Fast for at least eight hours before the test (you can drink water). The liver's job is to release stored sugar slowly over the periods when you are not eating. If your liver doesn't do its job, you get hangry. You'll know you have a problem if your blood sugar level is under 72 ng/mL or you run a hemoglobin A1C, and it shows that is too low or too high (anything below 4.2 or above 5.8 to 6.0). The hemoglobin A1C tests looks at how much damage sugar crystals in your blood are doing to your red blood cells over a three-month period. When your hemoglobin A1C is high, it means your average blood sugar content is at a point where it is likely damaging brain cells and the blood vessels in your body, especially the smaller vessels (like in the eyes and the kidneys). Poor blood sugar control greatly contributes to anxiety and poor mood. I see many patients whose anxiety relaxes when we get blood sugar in order.

Insulin is the hormone your pancreas secretes when you eat food. In fact, even the sight of food will cause our brain to send the signal to release insulin. The serum insulin test looks at how much insulin is around while you are in a fasting state. This number should normally be very low. If your insulin is high during a fasting state, you know that your pancreas is sending out more insulin than needed. High insulin levels will contribute to inflammation and poor mood, and indicate that your blood sugar may need more regulation. To fix blood sugar issues, refer to the blood sugar section in the last third of chapter 5.

CBC and Comp Metabolic Panel

These tests will check in on some basic systems in your body. The complete blood count (CBC) test looks at your red and white blood cells. Sometimes when red blood cells are low or white blood cells are unbalanced, anxiety can result. The complete metabolic panel (CMP) checks your liver, kidneys, and electrolytes. Abnormalities in any of these organ systems can contribute to mood changes and should be followed up with a physician.

Cholesterol Panel

While most doctors only worry about high cholesterol, I feel it is important to check for low cholesterol, too. Cholesterol is the building block for all steroid hormones, including ones that aid blood sugar regulation, blood pressure regulation, and proper sexual function. When your cholesterol is low, you are predisposed to anxiety.

Receptors are little docking stations where chemicals in the body connect to effect change in a cell. Cholesterol is crucial for the function of the receptors that work in the brain to recognize serotonin, the "feel-good" brain chemical that is often low in people with chronic anxiety. A fascinating study from 2010 looked at human cells treated with a statin medication. Statin drugs are the most prescribed drugs in the world. Researchers noted that the medication stopped the serotonin receptors from working properly, and only when extra cholesterol was added did these receptors start working again. Since the effect of serotonin is vitally important for good mood, it is important that cholesterol does not get too low. If you are predisposed to anxiety, you may want to be especially careful about using statins.

ABO Blood Type

You may already know your blood type, but did you know that blood type can predispose you to certain diseases and have an effect on how you respond to specific foods, even healthy choices? For example, people with blood type A may be more likely to have anxiety, while type Bs can have an inflammatory response to chicken. Learn more about this by reading Dr. Peter D'Adamo's book, *Eat Right for Your Type.* I have worked with the blood type diet in patients who did not respond to other diet plans. Running the ABO blood type, if you haven't done so already, will allow you to pursue this work further.

Inflammation Panel: Homocysteine, CRP, and Whole Blood Histamine

Homocysteine, C-reactive protein (CRP), and histamine are three tests that measure inflammation. As we have discussed, inflammation in the body and the brain will cause mood issues like anxiety by disrupting the ability of the nervous system to properly carry signals.

Imagine a pile of electrical wires with murky water thrown all over them—they probably don't work so well. Well, your nervous system is the same way—and when the nervous system is not working well, anxiety can result.

Homocysteine is an inflammatory molecule in the blood vessels typically associated with risk of heart disease. Animal studies link it to anxiety response as well. If your homocysteine levels are high, look for a special B vitamin formula that contains about 40 mg of vitamin B6, 1,000 mcg of vitamin B12, and about 1 gram of the methyltetrahydrofolate form of folate. Trimethylglycine is related to B vitamins and should be dosed at 3,600 mg every day. There are a number of supplements designed for homocysteine support. Choose one that includes all the above in one formula.

C-reactive protein is a marker of inflammation in the body that is probably a much better indicator of cardiovascular and heart disease risk than cholesterol. Even more pertinent to you, high CRP levels have been linked to generalized anxiety disorder. If your CRP levels are high, you can lower them by following the tips below.

Increase your fiber intake by adding 1 tsp of psyllium in a large glass of water once or twice a day

Add fish oil to your diet. About 1,000 mg of eicosapentaenoic acid (EPA) will modestly help.

Boost your vitamin C. A study from the University of California looked at almost four hundred smokers and found that 1,000 mg of vitamin C a day lowered their CRP by 25 percent.

Cut out fried foods and foods cooked at a high temperature. These are called advanced glycation endproducts (AGEs). A study on potato chip intake revealed that eating those delicious little chips for four weeks increased the oxidation of LDL and C-reactive protein levels. (See chapter 5 for more about AGEs.) Eating foods that are cooked at low temperature (soups, slow cooker, boiled foods, oatmeal) is better.

Increase your exercise. Interval training is best for this.

Like homocysteine, the whole blood histamine level test provides valuable information about how to use B vitamins to help to calm inflammation. Pioneers in the use of vitamins for mental health, such as Carl Pfeiffer and Bill Walsh, have used decades of clinical experience to figure out the histamine connection. People with high histamine (greater than 70) tend to have low neurotransmitter levels, which can contribute to anxiety.

If you have high histamine, try adding B vitamins, folate, and trimethylglycine to your diet. Patients with high histamine who also have hives and skin rashes will benefit from the bioflavonoid quercetin (250 mg, 3x/day) and vitamin C (500 mg, 3x/day).

If you have low histamine (below 40) you may need to avoid B vitamins and folate.

Iron Panel

The body needs iron in order to carry oxygen around. If a person who is predisposed to anxiety has low iron levels, he or she is more likely to suffer from anxiety. One 2013 study of school children with low iron levels found that a multiple vitamin with extra iron boosted the oxygen-carrying factor of the blood, hemoglobin, while reducing anxiety.

An iron panel includes serum iron, which tests the amount of iron traveling in the blood, and ferritin, which looks at iron storage. Many doctors do not run ferritin, so make sure yours does. Often a patient's serum iron will be normal but his ferritin is abysmally low, causing the body to stay in an anxiety state.

If your serum iron and/or ferritin are low, talk with your doctor. It is important to rule out any abnormal bleeding problems that can contribute to low numbers. To help raise iron levels, try the following ideas.

> Assure adequate iron intake. The best sources of absorbable iron are meats, like beef and dark turkey. If you are a vegetarian or vegan, use an iron skillet and eat plenty of dark green vegetables.

> Consider an iron supplement. A gentle supplement usually supplies about 25 mg per capsule, and I typically prescribe one to three capsules a day. The gentler forms of iron, succinate or fumarate, help prevent constipation. Taking iron with vitamin C (500 mg) will help absorption. Also, herbal nettles and yellow dock tea are good sources to support iron absorption.

Also, high levels of iron or ferritin can cause toxicity in the body. If these are high, work with a hematologist to look into possible reasons. Sometimes high ferritin can also suggest inflammation in the body.

Hormonal Panel

In this panel, we will look at a few hormonal regulators that can be factors in anxiety.

The thyroid panel includes TSH, free and total T3 (triiodothyronine) and T4 (thyroxine), and reverse T3. Typically, when levels of thyroid hormones T3 or T4 are high, patients can experience anxiety symptoms, especially heart palpitations, sweating, and tremors. Sounds a lot like anxiety, doesn't it? Patients with low T3 and T4 have reported weight loss, loose stools, and greasy skin. When thyroid hormone levels are high for a long time, patients can develop a bulging eye condition called exophthalmos. When thyroid levels are too high, the brain will shut down production of thyroid-stimulating hormone and you will see numbers around .02 microunits per milliliter (mcU/mL) or even lower.

When a patient is under high stress, his reverse T3 will be on the high end. This is because the body is using up its stores of T4. When reverse T3 goes up, regular T3 levels go down, causing fatigue.

If your T4 and/or T3 levels are high, talk to an endocrinologist (hormone specialist). Herbs like Melissa and motherwort can help calm the thyroid, but they should be used with the help of naturopathic doctor or other practitioner who is well trained and has checked out the reasons for the thyroid dysfunction.

Parathyroid (PTH)

Not well known, the four pea-sized parathyroid glands are located in the tissues of the thyroid. When PTH is high, this means these little guys are working too hard. High PTH can cause digestive issues, bone problems, high blood levels of calcium, and mood symptoms including anxiety, obsessive-compulsive disorder, depression, hostility, and even psychoticism. High PTH will also lower vitamin D levels, contributing to poor mood. Both depressive disorders and anxiety can normalize after treatment, which may include surgical removal of one or two of the four glands. While PTH is not routinely tested, it is worth checking if vitamin D is consistently low or if your calcium levels are high.

Serum Cortisol

Cortisol is one of the main stress hormones secreted by your adrenal gland. Cortisol helps the body fight stress, and it releases stored blood sugar from the liver. It is also responsible for balancing inflammation.

Cortisol naturally increases in the early morning hours to help us wake up, peaks around noon, and then decreases as the day goes along. At bedtime, it is usually quite low, and stays low until the early morning hours. Patients with acute anxiety often have high cortisol levels. The serum cortisol test should be taken in the morning (before 10:00 a.m., if possible), when cortisol is at its highest.

If your morning cortisol is above the normal range, there are a few steps you can take to stave off the morning "hit" of anxiety:

Go to bed at a reasonable and consistent time every night. In order to support regular circadian rhythms, it is important to have a ritual your body can count on.

If you are having sleeping problems, follow the recommendations in chapter 3.

It may be helpful to eat some food before bed. Try a protein and healthy carbohydrate snack, like a piece of turkey and some celery or even a rice cake with almond butter.

Try to get outside in the sunlight in the morning in order to help establish the optimal cortisol rhythm for the day.

The supplements phosphatidylserine, decapeptides (milk-derived amino acids), and fish oil can help balance cortisol. Start with 500 mg of phosphatidylserine before bedtime, and then add 175mg of the decapeptides. Also, 250 mg of magnesium glycinate before bedtime can be useful. It is best to start with one supplement for a night or two, and add the others one at a time after two days if you are not finding clear benefits with only one.

A 2003 study of diabetic patients showed how regular fish oil during the day, at a dose of 1,000 mg of eicosapentatoic acid (EPA), will balance cortisol in cases of chronic anxiety.

Meditation may be the most powerful way to lower excess cortisol. Regular practice is key. Find more about meditation in chapter 6.

After we discuss the rest of the below blood tests, we talk about a special saliva test that looks at cortisol levels over the course of the day.

Dehydroepiandroterone (DHEA) and Dehydroepiandroterone Sulfate (DHEAs)

Like cortisol, DHEA and its brother DHEAs are made by the adrenal glands. These two hormones play roles in inflammation, fertility, and thyroid hormone function. DHEA helps protect the nervous system—especially from the ravages of the stress hormone cortisol. As we age, DHEA naturally decreases, especially in those who do not exercise and keep mentally active.

DHEA can help soothe anxiety. A study of patients going through heroin withdrawal found that extra DHEA helped lower stress as the addicts weaned off the drug. Those who did not take the DHEA experienced much greater anxiety. Drug withdrawal causes some pretty serious anxiety, so if DHEA works on that, it will probably work in less serious cases.

It is helpful to check levels of DHEA and DHEAs in the blood. When these are high, the body is likely in an acute stress state. When they are low, it's likely that the person has been in a stress state for such a long time that the adrenals are starting to poop out. Low levels are associated with chronic anxiety and depression. This is known informally as "adrenal fatigue," a condition conventional medicine does not really recognize and sometimes holistic practitioners overemphasize. We will talk more about adrenal fatigue states when we discuss adrenal saliva testing.

If DHEA levels are high:

Start a meditation practice.

Begin an exercise regimen.

Consider an adaptogenic herb, like eleutherococcus, which balances the adrenal stress system.

If DHEA levels are low:

Meditation, good sleep, and exercise are important.

Consider supplemental DHEA. While supplemental DHEA is an over the counter supplement, it is still a hormone and should be used carefully and under the supervision of a knowledgeable practitioner. I generally start with 5 mg for women, and 15 mg for men. Once started, it is best to check blood and saliva levels every four to six weeks before increasing dose. If levels do not increase, then increase by increments of 5 mg in women and 10 mg in men, and recheck levels. Theoretically, there's a chance DHEA can push levels of other hormones like estrogen and testosterone, so if you have a risk or history of hormone-related cancers (such as breast, ovarian, or prostate cancer), you may want to consider other anxiety work or be extra vigilant with checking blood and saliva levels.

High levels of DHEA can cause increase facial and midline belly hair in women, and may also cause sweaty oily skin. The only food source of DHEA is the wild yam, but levels are too low for any clinical effect.

Testosterone: Free and Total

Known as the central male hormone, testosterone is known to help men with sexual drive and to avoid depression. But women need testosterone, too. Studies have shown that low levels of testosterone contribute to depression, low libido, and anxiety.

If testosterone is low, prioritize sleep—it's key for testosterone production. Also, start exercising and building muscle. Exercise sends signals the body to start making more testosterone to build more muscle. Consider testosterone-boosting herbs like horny goat weed (yes, that's a real herb), ashwagandha, and maca.

If these recommendations do not drive up your testosterone levels after three months, consider taking a prescription testosterone. While there are a number of forms available, I recommend a prescription transdermal (through the skin) patch. Transdermal patches get the horone into the body slowly and do less damage to the liver than oral and injectable administrations. Like DHEA above, too much testosterone can cause excess hair in the wrong places, acne, and changes in mood. People with hormonal cancer risks should be cautious with testosterone replacement. Interestingly, low testosterone has been associated with prostate cancer risk. Like anything else in life, you don't want to have too much or too little testosterone.

Serum Estrogen and Progesterone

As any woman who suffers from premenstrual moodiness may know too well, imbalances in female hormones undoubtedly play a role in mood.

Estrogen is the body's primary female hormone, and research shows how ups and downs in estrogen will change the levels of the feel-good neurotransmitter serotonin. Progesterone is a calming and relaxing hormone that also helps maintain GABA levels. The research on progesterone in women shows that it helps calm the brain, improve sleep, and even improve libido. One 2000 study from the Mayo Clinic looked at 176 post-menopausal women and found that when the women took oral micronized progesterone (a natural form of progesterone), they had much less body pain, fewer hot flashes, and less anxiety and depression. This study showed that the natural hormones did a better job than the medroxyprogesterone acetate (a synthetic progesterone) forms used in conventional gynecology practices. If you are interested in natural progesterone, ask your doctor for it. Otherwise, you will probably be prescribed the synthetic stuff, which has been associated with more side effects.

My takeaway from these hormonal studies is that hormonal replacement may help on the right person, but it's not for everyone. That's why this book covers foods, lifestyle, sleep, exercise, and nutritional supplementation, too—they are all part of a full approach that will work for your anxiety.

The best time to test estrogen is on the third day of menstrual flow; the best day to measure progesterone is day twenty-one of a woman's cycle. While it is inconvenient to have your blood taken on two separate days, this will give you the best indications of these hormone levels.

If Your Estrogen and/or Progesterone Is Low

As a point of caution, the use of any hormones, synthetic or natural, should not be taken casually. In fact, I do not recommend them until more basic care is performed first (such as balancing the diet, exercise, and sleep). In my experience with patients over the last decade, when these basics are addressed, women end up not needing additional hormones because the body is able to balance them on its own. In the small percentage where hormones are still needed, lower doses can achieve desired results.

If it still makes sense for you to try the hormones to help anxiety, consider natural hormone replacement therapy instead of conventional synthetic hormones. While there is less research on natural therapies, the studies that are available show that the side effects are fewer, for the body knows how to utilize the hormones over their synthetic sisters. With natural hormones, there are no strange metabolites produced—something that occurs with the fake stuff.

Progesterone itself may be most useful in cases where there is much anxiety and sleeplessness, especially in perimenopausal and menopausal women. While I generally recommend skin creams for hormone replacement, for cases of insomnia and anxiety, I suggest taking an oral dose (50–150 mg) of micronized progesterone at bedtime. This will raise GABA levels in the brain and help it relax.

When estrogen is low, consider estrogen treatments to help serotonin work its best. In addition to the estrogen, it's always a good idea to use some progesterone to protect the tissues in the body that may be susceptible to cancer risk (such as the breast and uterus).

Compounding pharmacies are the best source for natural hormones and will formulate them based on your specific needs. Natural hormones are prescribed as creams, oral preparations, or subdermal pellets, and can include estrogen, progesterone, testosterone, and DHEA.

Celiac Panel

Sometimes conventional doctors are puzzled when I recommend a celiac panel for my anxious patients. The conventional wisdom is that anxiety is a brain issue—why in the world would that crazy naturopath want to see a digestive test?

Here's the thing: when digestion is out of whack, the brain suffers. We talked about this in chapter 5.

Celiac is an immune reaction to the gluten part of wheat or spelt grains. One out of every hundred persons is affected. With skyrocketing grain intake over the last few decades, there's been a dramatic rise in celiac disease. Both celiac and nonceliac gluten sensitivity will contribute to mood disorders in adults and behavior problems in kids. While most people don't know they have it, one study shows that undiagnosed celiac poses a 400 percent increase risk of death overall—with those kinds of odds, I think a simple blood test is worth checking.

A celiac panel is made up of four different tests: antigliadin antibodies IgG, antigliadin antibodies IgM, Tissue Transglutamase (TTG), and secretory IgA. Together, these tests can help identify immune reactions to gluten about 90 percent of the time. The most accurate test is a biopsy (taking a piece of tissue from the small intestine). If you a going to get the blood test, make sure you are eating gluten regularly for at least four weeks before. Otherwise, you may not show up positive, even if you are.

What to Do if You Have Celiac Disease

Simply stated, it is best to avoid all gluten proteins, which occur in wheat, spelt, and amaranth products. When you go gluten-free, your gut wall linings typically heal within three to six months. In my clinical experience, mood issues will start to get better in as little as two to four weeks. While staying gluten-free, you should remember that grains like rice, quinoa, millet, and wild rice are perfectly fine to eat. Most oats are fine, too. Like any addictive drug, gluten withdrawal can be ugly, so remove it from your diet slowly, over a few weeks.

Even if you're not celiac positive, there still may be an advantage to going gluten free—read more about this in chapter 5.

Nutrient Panel

For all my patients, checking out nutrient levels is a must. While there are many to check, here are a few of my go-to tests that help identify the root causes of your anxiety.

Serum Carnitine

Serum carnitine is an amino acid that shuttles energy from the mitochondria out to the rest of the body. Mitochondria are the energy powerhouses in the cells, and they are prevalent in the nervous system, where neurotransmitters are made. Carnitine has been shown to lower inflammation and protect the nervous system from anxiety. In some patients who are low in carnitine, supplementing will reduce fatigue, which reduces anxiety.

Normal carnitine levels are usually between 28 and 60 micromoles per liter. If you are low, start with 500 mg of L-carnitine twice a day, preferably away from food for best absorption. Recheck carnitine blood levels in about six weeks; if there is no improvement, consider doses up to 3,000 mg per day and read up on digestive support. Sometimes, carnitine levels do rise because the digestive tract is not absorbing well. I have found raising carnitine to be extremely helpful, especially in women who experience anxiety issues after having a child.

The word *carnitine* comes from the Latin word *carne*, which means meat. It's no surprise that the highest concentrations of this amino acid are found in red meat. You can also find some carnitine in dairy products, nuts and seeds, and some beans, vegetables, and grains.

Serum Folic Acid and Serum B12

Known best for preventing the neurologic disorder spina bifida in newborns, folic acid also plays a key role in the production of the neurotransmitters dopamine, norepinephrine and epinephrine. Vitamin B12 is known to help support production of red blood cells and DNA, support nervous tissue, and play a role in normalizing pathways in the body that help with the production of serotonin and other neurotransmitters.

If your folic acid and/or B12 is low, take both folic acid (1,000 mcg or more) and oral vitamin B12 (1,000 mcg) daily. B vitamins like folic acid and B12 are water-soluble and generally safe. Methylcobalamin is the preferred form of vitamin B12. The methyltetrahydrofolate version of folic acid is the most natural form, while regular "folic acid" supplements should be avoided.

If your B12 and folic acid levels are normal but symptoms of anxiety are present, it may still be prudent to supplement with extra B12 and folic acid, especially if medication treatments are not working on their own.

Serum 25 (OH) Vitamin D

Known for helping keep bones healthy, vitamin D is actually a steroid molecule. When vitamin D is low, there is increased risk of virtually every disease: heart disease, cancer, autoimmune problems, and much more. I first learned about the benefits of vitamin D when I started doing depression research almost twenty years ago. I learned then that depressed patients typically have very low levels of vitamin D. Low vitamin D affects serotonin levels. As you probably already guessed, low vitamin D also contributes to anxiety, too.

Ranges between 30 to 100 ng/mL of vitamin D are normal in adults. An ideal level of vitamin D is around 50, and in my experience, very few patients with mood issues come in with healthy levels. Sunlight exposure is the method nature prescribed for humans to maintain vitamin D levels. There are very few vitamin D food sources, and eating large amounts of these are not really enough to raise levels of D once already low.

If your levels are low, start with a supplement, especially if you can't get out in the sun (see chapter 4 for info on safe sunning). The loose rule of thumb is to take about 2,000 IU per day of vitamin D3 for every 10 ng/mL you are looking to increase. For example, if a patient is at 20 ng/mL and I would like to see her levels at 50 ng/mL, then I will start with about 6,000 IU per day as a reasonable dose for three months.

The best dietary source of vitamin D is fish. Much of the literature ascribes the mood benefit of fish to its essential fatty acid content, but I believe that vitamin D also plays a role. Eggs, butter, mushrooms, and parsley have small amounts of D.

Vitamin D Toxicity: Vitamin D is a fat-soluble steroid molecule that can be toxic in high levels. Toxicity of vitamin D may lead to high calcium in the blood, kidney issues, and excessive bone loss. It is not known what supplemental amount may be problematic for a particular individual. Since this number may vary from patient to patient, it is best to run lab tests to check pre- and postsupplementation. As a guide, one 2009 study reviewed at the annual meeting of the American Academy of Neurology showed that patients given long-term treatment of 14,000 IU per day orally helped mood and had no toxicity. While I would not recommend you take doses this high without supervision, it gives you a sense of the safety of vitamin D.

There are two types of D on the market: D2 and D3. Plants manufacture vitamin D2 whereas vitamin D3 is synthesized by humans in the skin when it is exposed to UVB rays from sunlight. Clinically, I tend to use vitamin D3, which has been studied the most. If you are not finding benefit with vitamin D3, vitamin D2 may be a consideration for you.

Although there are a few forms of vitamin D in the body that can be tested, the test indicative of true vitamin D status is *25-hydroxy (OH) vitamin D*, and is the best to make clinical decisions regarding dosing.

Plasma Zinc and Serum Copper

Like lithium, zinc and copper are both trace minerals needed for emotional health. Zinc deficiency will contribute to emotional instability and anxiety. Zinc may also block the anxiety producing effects of glutamate, a neurotransmitter found naturally in the brain and in food additives (like monosodium glutamate, aka MSG).

Emerging information suggests that the relative amounts of zinc to copper may play a role in mood. Higher zinc-to-copper ratios are known to be predictive of good sleep, less insomnia, and less anxiety. A study from 2011 looked at thirty-eight people with anxiety as well as sixteen nonanxious individuals. It was shown that people with anxiety had much higher levels of copper relative to zinc and that zinc supplements helped normalize the ratios and reduce anxiety.

Another study looked at patients with anxiety with low zinc levels, especially in relationship to copper levels. In these patients, zinc piccolinate daily for eight weeks restored that balance and improved symptoms.

Normal zinc levels range between 0.66 and 1.10 mcg/mL. If your levels are below 0.9, and/or if your copper levels are in the high normal or above normal range, then start taking some zinc.

Optimal zinc dosage is 15 to 30 mg a day, taken with food. If your copper levels are normal and you are taking zinc for more than two months, take a milligram or two of copper every day—extra zinc can cause the body to lose copper. The top zinc sources include beef, lamb, turkey, chicken, pork, crabmeat, lobster, clams, and salmon. The best vegetable source is pumpkin seed.

Genetic Testing

The above tests were straight-on blood tests. The next two are genetic tests. These are a little more fancy and high-tech—they don't look at compounds in your blood, but rather at your genetic material—the book of life that includes all the information that makes you who you are. Genetic tests look your genes, the little codes that explain how to make something the cell needs to live.

Catechol-O-Methyltransferase (COMT)

COMT is a gene that codes for a protein enzyme that helps balance neurotransmitters. The effects of this are especially important in the prefrontal cortex of the brain, an area associated with the personality, thinking patterns, and emotions. People who have changes in this gene are much more likely to develop depression, anxiety, bipolar disorder, and even schizophrenia. Interestingly, they also have a higher disposition for temporomandibular joint disorder (known as TMJ). Not surprisingly, there is a strong association between anxiety and TMJ.

When there are abnormalities in this gene, dopamine and the stress hormone epinephrine do not get broken down properly, and you end up with way too much of each. This will create toxic metabolites like ammonia that cause more brain inflammation, and more anxiety.

As a result, people who have variations of the COMT gene experience anxiety and high startle responses. Generally, those with

COMT variation are like you—high-level thinkers with high levels of anxiety. It is possible that people with this genetic change may store higher levels of dopamine, epinephrine, and other neurotransmitters, which make a person less able to take his attention away from unpleasant pictures and sounds. Some are thrill seekers or gamblers. Oftentimes, these patients will not respond well to SSRI medications—which may make them worse, for increasing serotonin in the brain will only create more imbalances. Typically, they feel horrible when drinking coffee.

If your COMT is abnormal, balance your blood sugar (see above and chapter 5). Proper sugar and insulin levels go a long way to balance excess dopamine and epinephrine. Exercise (see chapter 4) will also help burn excess epinephrine. Eat lots of green vegetables and high antioxidant foods, like berries, red peppers, pomegranate, and goji berries. You can try antioxidant supplementation—n-acetyl cysteine is a precursor to glutathione, the master antioxidant in the body. Consider calming supplements like GABA (250 mg three times a day) and magnesium glycinate (250 mg once a day). Learn more about these supplements in chapter 7.

MTHFR Gene Test

Another relatively new genetic test is the methylenetetrahydrofolate reductase (whew, that's a mouthful) or MTHFR gene test. (The people who came up with that acronym must have been laughing all day in the lab. Work with this acronym however you would like!) Nevertheless, the MTHFR test is gaining attention in both holistic and conventional medical circles. This gene codes for an enzyme, methylenetetrahydrofolate reductase, that is needed to process folic acid into its most useful form, methyltetrahydrofolate (MTHF). Like COMT, this test checks for mutations in the gene.

MTHF has a strong link to both anxiety and depression. Abnormality in this gene make much harder for the body to produce neurotransmitters in proper balance.

If your MTHFR is abnormal, supplement with extra folate. The best form is methyltetrahydrofolate (MTHF), not regular folic acid. MTHF is often dosed anywhere from 1 to 5 mg a day, which is much higher than what is found in a multiple vitamin or even most prenatal vitamins. I usually recommend a starting dose of 1 mg a day of methylfolate. Eat green leafy vegetables for a natural source of methylfolate.

Salivary Adrenal Panel

There is one special test I like to run for patients who experience anxiety that doesn't involve blood. This one is even easier—it just involves a little spit.

The salivary adrenal panel is virtually ignored by the conventional medical community, but it is often run by naturopathic physicians and more holistically minded doctors. It measures your stress hormone, cortisol, at four points in the day: 6 a.m., 12 p.m., 6 p.m., and midnight. Earlier in this appendix, we talked about testing the blood for cortisol once, in the morning. I want to discuss why I like this saliva test even more.

The salivary adrenal panel can tell you whether your HPA stress system is running normal, too high, too low, or all over the place. If you don't remember the HPA stress system, give that section of chapter 2 a quick review right now.

This test will tell you if your brain's cerebral cortex is overtaxing your system and your adrenal glands are pumping excess cortisol and DHEA. Here is the normal cortisol range:

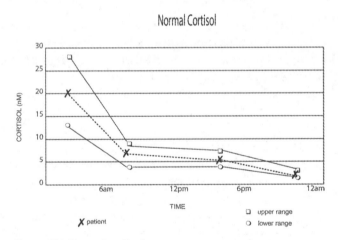

Figure A1.1: Normal cortisol

Your cortisol should be running somewhere in between the top and the bottom line throughout the day. If your stress system is running normal, your cortisol will be higher in the morning, come down during the day, and stay low until the morning hours. If the above figure is how your system looks with the test, then you can skip this section.

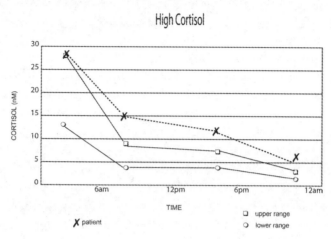

Figure A1.2: High cortisol

When your system is stressed out, you will see high cortisol, and it will look like Figure A1.2 above. Often, when you have undergone stress for a long time, your system is so depleted that your cortisol levels will be low all the time. I see this particular scenario often. It looks like this:

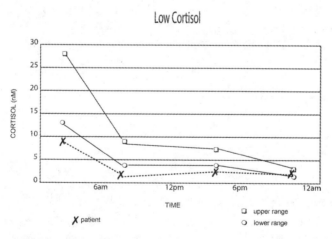

Figure A1.3: Low cortisol

Finally, there are people who have a mixed pattern, where it is up at certain times a day, and lower at other times a day.

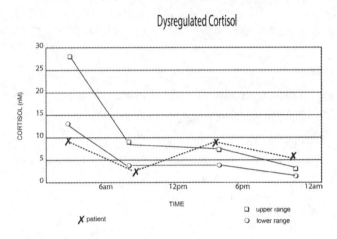

Figure A1.4: Dysregulated circadian cortisol

Fix Your Cortisol Patterns

No matter whether your cortisol is running high or low, the following steps will help you to normalize the levels.

1. Establish a proper sleep schedule and rhythm. Chapter 3 goes over exactly how to do this.

2. Eat at the same time of the day and do not eat a big meal too late. Cortisol rhythmicity is established by your eating patterns. Erratic eating times will help create erratic adrenal stress patterns.

3. If your schedule allows, try to get outside in the early morning after the sun comes up and exercise at least three days a week.

If you have high levels of cortisol, try these tips:

1. Follow the above recommendations for "all imbalance types."

2. Meditate and practice yoga. These are known to lower cortisol.

3. Take phosphatidylserine at 300 mg, three times a day. Phosphatidylserine supplementation has been shown to help lower cortisol.

4. Rhodiola: this botanical is an "adaptogen," which means when hormone levels are too high, it lowers them and when levels are too low, it can bring them

up. Taking 250 mg twice a day will help lower overall production of cortisol in response to stress. See chapter 6 for more about rhodiola.

5. Vitamin C with bioflavonoids: 500 mg three times a day. In one German study, good old vitamin C has also been shown to be a potent reducer of cortisol, high blood pressure, and overall stress. I use Thorne's vitamin C with bioflavonoids.

If you have low cortisol:

1. Follow the above recommendations for "all imbalance types."

2. Purchase a 10,000-lux light box to use in the morning for at least thirty minutes.

3. Start taking a half tsp of licorice extract in a little warm water first thing in the morning. Licorice contains a compound that allows you to retain the cortisol your body does make. I recommend Wise Woman Licorice extract.

4. Start taking an adrenal support. I recommend AdrenAssist, used by my Inner Source Health clinic. This formula is a TCM-inspired formula with cordyceps (a mushroom), vitamin B5, and some bovine adrenal gland. It also contains the herbal adaptogens ashwagandha and eleutherococcus. Start with one capsule in the morning and at midday for two weeks, then move to two capsules in the morning and midday.

If you have an imbalanced cortisol rhythm:

1. Follow the above recommendations for "all imbalance types."

2. Start taking the AdrenAssist formula mentioned above: one capsule in the morning and at midday.

3. Find the area of low cortisol and start taking the licorice mentioned above.

4. Find the area of high cortisol, and start taking two capsules of lactium casein decapeptide at that time. Lactium works pretty fast, helps decrease release of cortisol, calms the brain without sedating, and allows the brain to recognize cortisol more easily. When the brain can recognize cortisol, it doesn't send the signal to the adrenal gland to make more. Lactium is derived from casein, so anyone with a dairy allergy may need to be careful with it. I found good results using Sereniten by Douglas Labs

Check Your Pee: Urine Kryptopyrroles

Pyroluria (sometimes called malvaria) is caused by excessive levels of pyrroles. Dr. Abram Hoffer, a Canadian psychiatrist and biochemist, discovered that some of his patients with anxiety, depression, and mood swings had high amounts of something he called "the mauve factor" in their urine. This refers to excessive amounts of a molecule called kryptopyrrole, a byproduct of the adrenal gland that revs too high for too long. The pyrroles tend to attach to zinc, vitamin B6, manganese, and fatty acids (especially omega-6 and GLA) and usher them out of the body quickly, creating deficiencies. Hoffer found that when urine kryptopyrroles are high, these nutrients help the patient's mood. While this work has been largely ignored in modern psychiatry, in my clinical experience, I have seen a subset of patients for whom this is applicable, especially when adrenal testing is also showing cortisol levels to be high as well.

There is one laboratory online that I know offers this testing: *https://pyroluriatesting.com.*

Toxicity Blood Test Panel: GGT, Serum Metals (Lead, Mercury, Cadmium, Aluminum)

Toxins are everywhere. In 2009, the Centers for Disease Control looked at samples of blood and urine in 2,400 individuals. Researchers learned that most Americans have more than 212 toxins weighing them down—even newborn babies have them.

I look closely at environmental toxicity in my most difficult patients. I like to consider various toxins, which for the right person can contribute to or cause anxiety, depression, schizophrenia, bipolar, and many other mood symptoms. I call these psychiatrogens. Learn more about these psychiatrogens, how to test them, and how to treat them at *www.drpeterbongiorno.com/psychiatrogen.*

The first one of the toxicity tests, gamma-glutamyl transferase (GGT), looks at an enzyme that helps the liver recycle nutrients and antioxidants in its fight to detoxify the body. In conventional care, GGT is a biomarker used to check liver function. It is often considered an "alcoholic's blood test," for alcoholics typically have high GGT. But research shows that GGT is a pretty good way to tell about toxic body burden in general, including excess red meat consumption, heavy metals exposure, medication use, toxic herbs, and even breathable toxins like paint fumes and vinyl. GGT levels near the high of 40 have been associated with increased rates of diabetes and heart disease.

The most common heavy metal culprits are lead, mercury, cadmium, and aluminum. Regarding these heavy metals, blood tests only tell us about very recent toxin exposure. If they are positive, then looking for the source is extremely valuable—for example, the water you are drinking, excessive amounts of high mercury fishes, or regular exposure to vehicle exhaust.

Hair Analysis and Urine Testing

If blood tests are negative, but my patients are not improving when using the other recommendations we already talked about, and/or something about their history suggests there may still be a toxicity picture, then the next step is to do hair analysis and urine tests, which can tell if the body took in toxins and stored them in places like the brain. Your naturopathic physician can run hair analysis and urine tests.

Hair analysis can help show exposure to chemicals, like heavy metals, that accumulate over several months. I like to use hair analysis as an indicator for possible low levels of lithium. It is a pretty straightforward test—clip some hair (usually at the nape of your neck), seal it in a plastic bag, and send it along for analysis. Two companies that run hair analysis are *www.traceelements.com* and *www.doctorsdata.com/hair-elements*.

Sometimes I will also look at urine testing of heavy metals and certain other toxins. A good company for urine testing is *www.doctorsdata.com*. Heavy metals deplete antioxidants in the body and damage the reuptake proteins the brain uses to remove glutamate (a common excitatory toxin the brain normally makes), thus rendering the brain cells damaged and inflamed. Excess brain inflammation contributes to anxiety and likely messes up brain serotonin, too. In a cyclic fashion, inflammation makes brain cells more vulnerable to toxins, which causes more anxiety.

heavy metals toxins ➞ brain inflammation ➞ anxiety

Heavy metals also contribute to anxiety by inhibiting the COMT enzyme we discussed earlier. Evidence suggests that mercury will also inactivate the methionine pathway, which is needed to produce healthy neurotransmitter levels. If your toxins or metal levels are high, good first steps to take include:

1. Make sure you are pooping every day. Elimination through the bowels is critical in order for your body to rid itself of toxins. You can start by adding plenty of water

(at least 60 ounces per day). Add high-fiber foods to your diet (like prunes, flax meal, apples, and oatmeal). Next, add 1 tsp of psyllium in the morning with a big glass of water.

2. Sweat it up with sauna and exercise. When you sweat, your body's elimination systems clean out and detoxify. Regular exercise is key. Use a sauna for ten minutes three times a week to increase the elimination. Remember, if you are sweating, you need to keep drinking water.

3. Add cilantro and chlorella. Cilantro is a beautiful herb that has the ability to gently release metals and toxins, and chlorella is a blue-green algae that helps move waste out of the body. Taking these together will gently release toxins from the tissue and move them out of the body. Start with 30 drops of cilantro tincture and 1 tsp of chlorella once a day; in two weeks, increase to twice a day. Do this for one month.

While these are helpful, sometimes more advanced protocols like chelation may be useful. The chelation process uses an oral or intravenous supplement to pull metals out of the body tissues. Chelation should only be done by a qualified practitioner. Ask your doctor if chelation may be necessary. In my experience, most patients who follow the above advice start to feel better and do not necessarily need to move on to chelation therapy.

Mold Testing

Many patients with anxiety are genetically susceptible to the toxins carried on various molds to which they may be exposed. These molds are present in houses, workplaces, and even on airplanes, trains, and public places that are not well ventilated or cleaned. Blood tests called an HLA DR panel can help identify whether you are susceptible to mold. When a person is susceptible to mold, their system will react with a lot of inflammation, which will contribute to anxiety or mood problems. A great book by a pioneer on the subject is *Mold Warriors* by Dr. Ritchie Shoemaker.

great natural medicine resources

There's a whole lot of information about natural health out there. Unfortunately, you cannot always trust it. Sometimes the science isn't very strong, or the motivation is more about money than health. The below list represents the best places to find good information and the right practitioners.

Naturopathic Physicians and Naturopathic Medicine

Naturopathic doctors (NDs) are trained in postcollege four-year medical programs. NDs learn all basics of primary care medicine at the same level as conventional medical doctors (MDs). NDs learn about anatomy, physiology, biochemistry, physical exams, minor surgery, blood draws, pharmacology (the study of medications), and so on. In a naturopathic curriculum, there is a much greater emphasis on holistic primary care experience with patients one on one and much less experience in hospitals and urgent care situations. Beyond conventional medical care, NDs learn a great deal about food, diet, exercise, nutrient therapies, and herbal medicines. The underlying tenet is to help the body to heal itself using the most natural means possible.

Naturopathic doctors are the perfect primary care physicians. Since there is a shortage of primary care doctors, naturopaths are needed more than ever. In Canada, Europe, and Australia, naturopathic doctors are licensed to practice medicine. In the US, naturopathic physicians are licensed to practice medicine in eighteen states and the District of Columbia. In those states, we practice as primary care physicians.

I am president of the New York State Association of Naturopathic Physicians. In our particular state, NDs are not licensed as physicians (even though our Connecticut neighbor to the north has been licensed since 1922), but we are actively pursuing our medical licenses. It seems in our state, and many others, the conventional society of medical doctors would prefer we do not have licenses. I think they feel threatened that we may take away their business. Given the shortage of primary care doctors, and given the sense of abundance in the world, we know that there are plenty of patients—so my hope is, in time, the public in all states, including New York, will have the choice of seeing a naturopathic physician as their primary care doctor. Please visit *www.NYANP.org* and *www.naturopathic.org* to learn more about supporting NDs, so everyone can choose a naturopathic doctor for their healthcare.

Naturopathic Physicians

American Association of Naturopathic Physicians (AANP)
www.naturopathic.org
Founded in 1985, the American Association of Naturopathic Physicians (AANP) is the national professional society representing licensed naturopathic physicians. If you are looking to find a naturopathic doctor in your area, visit this website. Beware: many people call themselves naturopathic physicians, but do not have full medical training (many have online degrees). Some of these practitioners may have valuable information to offer you, but if you are looking for someone who also has medical training, use the AANP directory.

The American Holistic Medical Association
www.holisticmedicine.org
The American Holistic Medical Association (AHMA) was founded in July 1978 by medical doctors who had an interest in natural and holistic medicine but had virtually no support from their medical community. Today, members include medical doctors, naturopathic doctors, and many other practitioners. The AHMA runs excellent conferences, continuing education events, retreats, and are a source of community for the holistic medical profession.

The Institute of Functional Medicine (IFM)
www.functionalmedicine.org
IFM consists of medical doctors, osteopathic physicians, and naturopathic doctors who support a systems-based approach. Besides having a practitioner base, they also offer resources and conferences geared toward medical doctors and other conventional practitioners interested in learning more about holistic approaches.

Cognitive Behavioral Therapists

Anxiety and Depression Association of America
www.adaa.org

Acupuncturists

National Certification Commission for Acupuncture and Oriental Medicine
www.nccaom.org
This is the national certifying body for licensed acupuncturists. If you cannot find your acupuncturist's name here, you need to question whether he or she has been through the proper training.

Blood Type Diet

Eat Right for Your Blood Type
By Peter D'Adamo, with Catherine Witney
This is a landmark work from the mid-1990s that has helped millions figure out the best ways to use healthy foods to heal the body and mind. The original book is still printed in hardcover—a testament to its longevity.

Massage Therapists

The American Massage Therapy Association (AMTA)
www.amtamassage.org
This is the association for licensed massage therapists.

The National Certification Board for Therapeutic Massage & Bodywork (NCBTMB)
www.ncbtmb.org
This organization approves and board certifies massage therapists.

Homeopaths

American Institute of Homeopathy (AIH)

www.homeopathyusa.org

Established in 1844, the American Institute of Homeopathy is the oldest national US medical organization. Its members are licensed medical and osteopathic physicians, dentists, advanced practice nurses, and physician assistants who practice homeopathy. According to their website, the AIH strives to promote the public acceptance of homeopathy while safeguarding the interests of the profession.

Homeopathic Academy of Naturopathic Physicians (HANP)

www.hanp.net

This is a specialty society within the profession of naturopathic medicine. Naturopathic physicians with a strong interest in homeopathy often go for increased education and certification through this academy.

Inner Source Natural Health

www.InnerSourceHealth.com

This is the information for the New York clinic of Dr. Peter Bongiorno and Dr. Pina LoGiudice. Dr. LoGiudice is also a well-known naturopathic physician in her own right, having been called a "world expert" by Dr. Mehmet Oz after her first appearance on his show in June 2011.

Please sign up for the free Inner Source newsletter, which contains the latest information regarding research, natural medicine, and health.

Light Boxes

Verilux HappyLight

Northern Light Technologies Travelite

Carex Daylight Classic (DL930)

supplement resources

Assuring that you are taking high-quality supplements is very important, but regulation is unfortunately not very good at this time. The supplements mentioned below are used in our clinic and in the clinics of physicians who search for the highest quality supplements available. These are all allergen-free and are rigorously tested for contaminants, toxins, and chemicals.

www.3UNEED.com
This website supplies the same high quality, physician-grade basic multiple vitamins, fish oil, and probiotics. (I take them myself.) These vitamins are all-natural and contain no glutens, allergens, dairy components, or artificial colors or flavorings. They are also highly tested to be free of contaminants, pesticides, and heavy metals.

Source I and II Nutrients
A blend of the highest quality multiple vitamins and minerals

Ultimate Omega Fish Oil
An excellent, molecularly distilled essential fatty acid

Restoraflora Probiotic
Lactobacillus and bifidus combination, used to support optimal neurotransmitter health

AdrenAssist
A Chinese medicine–inspired formulation to support health adrenal function

Melatonin Cadence
A special time-release formula of melatonin to help naturally support optimal sleep

Tryptophan Calmplete
A blend of tryptophan and B vitamins to support serotonin for healthy sleep

Inner Source Health supplements are also available at the natural health store on *www.InnerSourceHealth.com.*

Licorice solid extract, by Wise Woman Herbals:
www.wisewomanherbals.com

Vitamin C with bioflavonoids, by Thorne Research: *www.thorne.com*

Sereniten, by Douglas Labs: *www.douglaslabs.com*

Seriphos, by Interplexus: *www.interplexus.com*

Robert's Formula, by Integrative Therapeutics: *www.integrativepro.com*

PheniTropic, by Biotics: *www.bioticsnw.com*

quick breakfast ideas

Poached Eggs on Sprouted Bread

Add one and a half inches of water to a deep pan and bring to a simmer. Swirl the water in a whirlpool fashion while quickly cracking and adding the first egg to the water. Then add the second egg. Cover the pan, turn off the heat, and let poach for five minutes—no peeking. While the eggs are poaching, toast two pieces of sprouted wheat bread. Butter the bread with organic butter, drain the eggs using a slotted spoon, then place them on the bread. You can also place an egg in ice water and save in the fridge for up to six hours.

Quick Oatmeal

Purchase organic quick oats. For each serving, place a half cup of oats in one cup of water. If you like it creamier, also add a half cup of almond milk per serving. Cook on low heat, and add one teaspoon of cinnamon, half a teaspoon of ghee, a handful of walnuts, a dash of salt, and half an apple, chopped well. Keep stirring while cooking to avoid sticking. Serve when cooked to the doneness you like. Add blueberries on top. Serve with a cup of fresh green tea.

Nut Butter on Sprouted Toast

Toast two slices of sprouted wheat bread. Then spread sunflower butter, raw almond butter, pumpkin butter, or other nut butter on the bread. Serve with a cup of fresh green tea.

Inner Source Cleanse Smoothie

In a blender, combine one scoop of Inner Source Cleanse powder (find it at *www.3UNeed.com*) or other healthy rice- or pea-based protein (about 18 grams) with four ounces of water or coconut milk, a handful of ice, a quarter cup of frozen organic blueberries, a quarter cup of frozen organic strawberries, and half a frozen banana. If you do not have a protein powder, you can add two tablespoons of almond butter instead.

Greek Yogurt Sundae
Mix six ounces of yogurt with a handful of walnuts and sunflower seeds and a handful of blueberries. Enjoy!

Dr. Peter's Gluten-Free Waffles
For three to four servings, combine two cups of gluten-free flour, one teaspoon of baking soda, one teaspoon of cinnamon, and a tablespoon of flax seeds. Then add two lightly beaten eggs, one teaspoon of vanilla extract, two-thirds of a stick of salted butter, a half cup of vanilla yogurt, and a cup of almond milk, then mix. Fold in a half cup of chopped pecans or other nuts.

Preheat your waffle maker while letting the batch sit for five minutes. Add batter to waffle maker and cook.

* You can make this dairy-free by removing the yogurt and adding another half cup of almond milk.
** You can make this breakfast more protein-rich by adding two tablespoons of rice protein powder and removing two tablespoons of gluten-free flour.

Look for more breakfast recipes at *www.drpeterbongiorno.com/breakfast*

references

Chapter 2

Bongiorno, Peter. "Stress, fear, trauma, and distress." In *Integrative Medicine for Depression,* eds. Brogan and Greenblatt. CRC Press, 2015.

Chapter 3

Abbasi, Behnood, Masud Kimiagar, Khosro Sadeghniiat, Minoo M. Shirazi, Mehdi Hedayati, and Bahram Rashidkhani. "The effect of magnesium supplementation on primary insomnia in elderly: a double-blind placebo-controlled clinical trial." *Journal of Research in Medical Sciences: The Official Journal of Isfahan University of Medical Sciences* 17, no. 12 (2012): 1161.

Centers for Disease Control and Prevention (CDC). "Insufficient sleep is a public health epidemic." (2013). *http://www.cdc.gov/features/dssleep/.*

Cohen, Sheldon, William J. Doyle, C. M. Alper, Denise Janicki-Deverts, and Ronald B. Turner. "Sleep habits and susceptibility to the common cold." *Archives of Internal Medicine* 169, no. 1 (2009): 62–67.

Fernández-San-Martín, Ma Isabel, Roser Masa-Font, Laura Palacios-Soler, Pilar Sancho-Gómez, Cristina Calbó-Caldentey, and Gemma Flores-Mateo. "Effectiveness of Valerian on insomnia: a meta-analysis of randomized placebo-controlled trials." *Sleep Medicine* 11, no. 6 (2010): 505–511.

Kripke, Daniel F., Robert D. Langer, and Lawrence E. Kline. "Hypnotics' association with mortality or cancer: a matched cohort study." *BMJ Open* 2, no. 1 (2012): e000850.

Murck, Harald. "Ketamine, magnesium, and major depression—from pharmacology to pathophysiology and back." *Journal of Psychiatric Research*: 955–65.

Rondanelli, Mariangela, Annalisa Opizzi, Francesca Monteferrario, Neldo Antoniello, Raffaele Manni, and Catherine Klersy. "The effect of melatonin, magnesium, and zinc on primary insomnia in long-term care facility residents in Italy: a double-blind, placebo-controlled clinical trial." *Journal of the American Geriatrics Society* 59, no. 1 (2011): 82–90.

Shen, Jianhua, Sidney H. Kennedy, Robert D. Levitan, Leonid Kayumov, and Colin M. Shapiro. "The effects of nefazodone on women with seasonal affective disorder: clinical and polysomnographic analyses." *Journal of Psychiatry and Neuroscience* 30, no. 1 (2005): 11.

Toffol, E., N. Kalleinen, J. Haukka, O. Vakkuri, T. Partonen, and P. Polo-Kantola. "Melatonin in perimenopausal and postmenopausal women." *Menopause* 1, no. 1.

Wesensten, Nancy Jo, Thomas J. Balkin, Rebecca M. Reichardt, Mary A. Kautz, George A. Saviolakis, and Gregory Belenky. "Daytime sleep and performance following a zolpidem and melatonin cocktail." *Sleep* 28, no. 1 (2005): 93–103.

Chapter 4

Babyak, Michael, James A. Blumenthal, Steve Herman, Parinda Khatri, Murali Doraiswamy, Kathleen Moore, W. Edward Craighead, Teri T. Baldewicz, and K. Ranga Krishnan. "Exercise treatment for major depression: maintenance of therapeutic benefit at 10 months." *Psychosomatic Medicine* 62, no. 5 (2000): 633–638.

Blumenthal, James A., Michael A. Babyak, Kathleen A. Moore, W. Edward Craighead, Steve Herman, Parinda Khatri, Robert Waugh et al. "Effects of exercise training on older patients with major depression." *Archives of Internal Medicine* 159, no. 19 (1999): 2349–2356.

Erickson, Kirk I., Michelle W. Voss, Ruchika Shaurya Prakash, Chandramallika Basak, Amanda Szabo, Laura Chaddock, Jennifer S. Kim, et al. "Exercise training increases size of hippocampus and improves memory." *Proceedings of the National Academy of Sciences* (2011): 201015950.

Schoenfeld, Brad Jon, Alan Albert Aragon, and James W. Krieger. "The effect of protein timing on muscle strength and hypertrophy: a meta-analysis." *Journal of the International Society of Sports Medicine* 10, no. 1 (2013): 53.

Santarelli, Luca, Michael Saxe, Cornelius Gross, Alexandre Surget, Fortunato Battaglia, Stephanie Dulawa, Noelia Weisstaub, et al. "Requirement of hippocampal neurogenesis for the behavioral effects of antidepressants." *Science* 301, no. 5634 (2003): 805–809.

Chapter 5

Addolorato, et al. "State and trait anxiety and depression in patients affected by gastrointestinal diseases: psychometric evaluation of 1641 patients referred to an internal medicine outpatient setting." *International Journal of Clinical Practice* 62, no. 7 (2008): 1063–1069.

Barbara, Giovanni, Lisa Zecchi, Raffaella Barbaro, Cesare Cremon, Lara Bellacosa, Marco Marcellini, Roberto De Giorgio, Roberto Corinaldesi, and Vincenzo Stanghellini. "Mucosal permeability and immune activation as potential therapeutic targets of probiotics in irritable bowel syndrome." *Journal of Clinical Gastroenterology* 46 (2012): S52–S55.

Bravo, Javier A., Paul Forsythe, Marianne V. Chew, Emily Escaravage, Hélène M. Savignac, Timothy G. Dinan, John Bienenstock, and John F. Cryan. "Ingestion of Lactobacillus strain regulates emotional behavior and central GABA receptor expression in a mouse via the vagus nerve." *Proceedings of the National Academy of Sciences* 108, no. 38 (2011): 16050–16055.

Butchko, Harriett H., W. Wayne Stargel, C. Phil Comer, Dale A. Mayhew, Christian Benninger, George L. Blackburn, Leo MJ de Sonneville, et al. "Aspartame: review of safety." *Regulatory Toxicology and Pharmacology* 35, no. 2 (2002): S1–S93.

Campanella, Jonia, Federico Biagi, Paola Ilaria Bianchi, Giovanni Zanellati, Alessandra Marchese, and Gino Roberto Corazza. "Clinical response to gluten withdrawal is not an indicator of coeliac disease." *Scandinavian Journal of Gastroenterology* 43, no. 11 (2008): 1311–1314.

Catassi, Carlo, Julio C. Bai, Bruno Bonaz, Gerd Bouma, Antonio Calabrò, Antonio Carroccio, Gemma Castillejo, et al. "Non-celiac gluten sensitivity: the new frontier of gluten related disorders." *Nutrients* 5, no. 10 (2013): 3839–3853.

dos Santos Vaz, Juliana, Gilberto Kac, Pauline Emmett, John M. Davis, Jean Golding, and Joseph R. Hibbeln. "Dietary patterns, n-3 fatty acids intake from seafood and high levels of anxiety symptoms during pregnancy: findings from the Avon Longitudinal Study of Parents and Children." *PloS One* 8, no. 7 (2013): e67671.

Hoch, Tobias, Silke Kreitz, Andreas Hess, and Monika Pischetsrieder. "Everyday desire: influence of snack food on whole brain activity patterns." In *Abstracts of Papers of the American Chemical Society*, vol. 245.

Jacka, Felice N., Simon Overland, Robert Stewart, Grethe S. Tell, Ingvar Bjelland, and Arnstein Mykletun. "Association between magnesium intake and depression and anxiety in community-dwelling adults: the Hordaland Health Study." *Australian and New Zealand Journal of Psychiatry* 43, no. 1 (2009): 45–52.

Lucas, Michel, Fariba Mirzaei, An Pan, Olivia I. Okereke, Walter C. Willett, Éilis J. O'Reilly, Karestan Koenen, and Alberto Ascherio. "Coffee, caffeine, and risk of depression among women." *Archives of Internal Medicine* 171, no. 17 (2011): 1571–1578.

Maes, Michael, P. C. D'haese, Simon Scharpé, Peter D'Hondt, P. Cosyns, and M. E. De Broe. "Hypozincemia in depression." *Journal of Affective Disorders* 31, no. 2 (1994): 135–140.

Miazga, Angelika, Maciej Osiński, Wojciech Cichy, and Ryszard Żaba. "Current views on the etiopathogenesis, clinical manifestation, diagnostics, treatment and correlation with other nosological entities of SIBO." *Advances in Medical Sciences* (2014).

Roberts, Hyman J. "Reactions attributed to aspartame-containing products: 551 cases." *Journal of Applied Nutrition* 40, no. 8 (1988): 5–94.

Rowe, Katherine S., and Kenneth J. Rowe. "Synthetic food coloring and behavior: a dose response effect in a double-blind, placebo-controlled, repeated-measures study." *The Journal of Pediatrics* 125, no. 5 (1994): 691–698.

Sánchez-Villegas, Almudena, Miguel Delgado-Rodríguez, Alvaro Alonso, Javier Schlatter, Francisca Lahortiga, Lluis Serra Majem, and Miguel Angel Martinez-Gonzalez. "Association of the Mediterranean dietary pattern with the incidence of depression: the Seguimiento Universidad de Navarra/University of Navarra follow-up (SUN) cohort." *Archives of General Psychiatry* 66, no. 10 (2009): 1090–1098.

Sturniolo, Giacomo C., Vincenza Di Leo, Antonio Ferronato, Anna D'Odorico, and Renata D'Incà. "Zinc supplementation tightens 'leaky gut' in Crohn's disease." *Inflammatory Bowel Diseases* 7, no. 2 (2001): 94–98.

Sturtzel, B., C. Mikulits, C. Gisinger, and I. Elmadfa. "Use of fiber instead of laxative treatment in a geriatric hospital to improve the wellbeing of seniors." *JNHA-The Journal of Nutrition, Health and Aging* 13, no. 2 (2009): 136–139.

Wong, M. L., and P. B. Bongiorno. "Interleukin (IL) 1b, IL-1 receptor antagonist, IL-b, and IL-13 gene expression in the central nervous system and anterior pituitary during systemic inflammation: pathophysiological implications." *Proceedings of the National Academy of Sciences* 94 (1997): 227–232.

Yoto, A., S. Murao, M. Motoki, Y. Yokoyama, N. Horie, K. Takeshima, K. Masuda, M. Kim, and H. Yokogoshi. "Oral intake of γ-aminobutyric acid affects mood and activities of central nervous system during stressed condition induced by mental tasks." *Amino Acids* 43, no. 3 (2012): 1331–1337.

Chapter 6

Brown, Marie-Annette, Jamie Goldstein-Shirley, Jo Robinson, and Susan Casey. "The effects of a multi-modal intervention trial of light, exercise, and vitamins on women's mood." *Women & Health* 34, no. 3 (2001): 93–112.

Chiesa, Alberto, and Alessandro Serretti. "Mindfulness-based stress reduction for stress management in healthy people: a review and meta-analysis." *The Journal of Alternative and Complementary Medicine* 15, no. 5 (2009): 593–600.

Cromie, William J. "Meditation found to increase brain size." *Harvard University Gazette* 23 (2006).

Field, Tiffany, Maria Hernandez-Reif, Miguel Diego, Saul Schanberg, and Cynthia Kuhn. "Cortisol decreases and serotonin and dopamine increase following massage therapy." *International Journal of Neuroscience* 115, no. 10 (2005): 1397–1413.

Fitzgerald, B. "Social media is causing anxiety, study finds." *http://www.huffingtonpost.com/2012/07/10/social-media-anxiety_n_1662224.html*

Hofmann, Stefan G., Alice T. Sawyer, Ashley A. Witt, and Diana Oh. "The effect of mindfulness-based therapy on anxiety and depression: a meta-analytic review." *Journal of Consulting and Clinical Psychology* 78, no. 2 (2010): 169.

Kirkwood, Graham, Hagen Rampes, Veronica Tuffrey, Janet Richardson, and Karen Pilkington. "Yoga for anxiety: a systematic review of the research evidence." *British Journal of Sports Medicine* 39, no. 12 (2005): 884–891.

Kooser, A. "Something new to fear: cell phone separation anxiety." *http://www.cnet.com/news/something-new-to-fear-cell-phone-separation-anxiety/*

Kutner, Jean S., Marlaine C. Smith, Lisa Corbin, Linnea Hemphill, Kathryn Benton, B. Karen Mellis, Brenda Beaty, et al. "Massage therapy versus simple touch to improve pain and mood in patients with advanced cancer: a randomized trial." *Annals of Internal Medicine* 149, no. 6 (2008): 369–379.

Li, Q., K. Morimoto, A. Nakadai, H. Inagaki, M. Katsumata, T. Shimizu, Y. Hirata, et al. "Forest bathing enhances human natural killer activity and expression of anti-cancer proteins." *International Journal of Immunopathology and Pharmacology* 20, no. 2 Suppl 2 (2006): 3–8.

Malenbaum, Sara, Francis J. Keefe, Amanda Williams, Roger Ulrich. "Effects of exposure to nature and abstract pictures on patients recovering from heart surgery." *Psychophysiology* 30 (Supplement 1, 1993): 7.

Mandal, Ananya. "Anxiety and depression linked to computer games." *http://www.news-medical.net/news/20120110/Anxiety-and-depression-linked-to-computer-games.aspx*

Mao, Gen-Xiang, Yong-Bao Cao, Xiao-Guang Lan, Zhi-Hua He, Zhuo-Mei Chen, Ya-Zhen Wang, Xi-Lian Hu, Yuan-Dong Lv, Guo-Fu Wang, and Jing Yan. "Therapeutic effect of forest bathing on human hypertension in the elderly." *Journal of Cardiology* 60, no. 6 (2012): 495–502.

Michalsen, Andreas, Paul Grossman, Ayhan Acil, Jost Langhorst, Rainer Lüdtke, Tobias Esch, George Stefano, and Gustav Dobos. "Rapid stress reduction and anxiolysis among distressed women as a consequence of a three-month intensive yoga program." *American Journal of Case Reports* 11, no. 12 (2005): CR555–CR561.

Moyer, Christopher A., James Rounds, and James W. Hannum. "A meta-analysis of massage therapy research." *Psychological Bulletin* 130, no. 1 (2004): 3.

Ornish, Dean, Jue Lin, June M. Chan, Elissa Epel, Colleen Kemp, Gerdi Weidner, Ruth Marlin, et al. "Effect of comprehensive lifestyle changes on telomerase activity and telomere length in men with biopsy-proven low-risk prostate cancer: 5-year follow-up of a descriptive pilot study." *The Lancet Oncology* 14, no. 11 (2013): 1112–1120.

Ornish, Dean, Larry W. Scherwitz, James H. Billings, K. Lance Gould, Terri A. Merritt, Stephen Sparler, William T. Armstrong, et al. "Intensive lifestyle changes for reversal of coronary heart disease." *JAMA* 280, no. 23 (1998): 2001–2007.

Park, Seong-Hyun, and Richard H. Mattson. "Ornamental indoor plants in hospital rooms enhanced health outcomes of patients recovering from surgery." *The Journal of Alternative and Complementary Medicine* 15, no. 9 (2009): 975–980.

Peterson, Linda Gay, and Lori Pbert. "Effectiveness of a meditation-based stress reduction program in the treatment of anxiety disorders." *American Journal of Psychiatry* 149 (1992): 936–943.

Pilkington, Karen, Graham Kirkwood, Hagen Rampes, Mike Cummings, and Janet Richardson. "Acupuncture for anxiety and anxiety disorders: a systematic literature review." *Acupuncture in Medicine* 25, no. 1–2 (2007): 1–10.

Samuels, Noah, Cornelius Gropp, Shepherd Roee Singer, and Menachem Oberbaum. "Acupuncture for psychiatric illness: a literature review." *Behavioral Medicine* 34, no. 2 (2008): 55–64.

Shannahoff-Khalsa, David S., Leslie E. Ray, S. Levine, C. C. Gallen, Barry J. Schwartz, and John J. Sidorowich. "Randomized controlled trial of yogic meditation techniques for patients with obsessive-compulsive disorder." *CNS Spectrums* 4, no. 12 (1999): 34–47.

Shokouhi-Moqhaddam, Solmaz, Noshiravan Khezri-Moghadam, Zeinab Javanmard, Hassan Sarmadi-Ansar, Mehran Aminaee, Majid Shokouhi-Moqhaddam, and Mahmoud Zivari-Rahman. "A study of the correlation between computer games and adolescent behavioral problems." *Addiction & Health* 5, no. 1–2 (2013): 43.

Streeter, Chris C., Theodore H. Whitfield, Liz Owen, Tasha Rein, Surya K. Karri, Aleksandra Yakhkind, Ruth Perlmutter, et al. "Effects of yoga versus walking on mood, anxiety, and brain GABA levels: a randomized controlled MRS study." *The Journal of Alternative and Complementary Medicine* 16, no. 11 (2010): 1145–1152.

Ulrich, Roger. "View through a window may influence recovery." *Science* 224, no. 4647 (1984): 224–225.

Wang, Hao, Hong Qi, Bai-song Wang, Yong-yao Cui, Liang Zhu, Zheng-xing Rong, and Hong-zhuan Chen. "Is acupuncture beneficial in depression? A meta-analysis of 8 randomized controlled trials." *Journal of Affective Disorders* 111, no. 2 (2008): 125–134.

Witt, Claudia M., Daniel Pach, Benno Brinkhaus, Katja Wruck, Brigitte Tag, Sigrid Mank, and Stefan N. Willich. "Safety of acupuncture: results of a prospective observational study with 229,230 patients and introduction of a medical information and consent form." *Forschende Komplementärmedizin/Research in Complementary Medicine* 16, no. 2 (2009): 91–97.

Chapter 7

"Practice guideline for the treatment of patients with major depressive disorder." American Psychiatric Association, 2010.

Akhondzadeh, Shahin, H. R. Naghavi, M. Vazirian, A. Shayeganpour, H. Rashidi, and M. Khani. "Passionflower in the treatment of generalized anxiety: a pilot double-blind randomized controlled trial with oxazepam." *Journal of Clinical Pharmacy and Therapeutics* 26, no. 5 (2001): 363–367.

Basselin, Mireille, Hyung-Wook Kim, Mei Chen, Kaizong Ma, Stanley I. Rapoport, Robert C. Murphy, and Santiago E. Farias. "Lithium modifies brain arachidonic and docosahexaenoic metabolism in rat lipopolysaccharide model of neuroinflammation." *Journal of Lipid Research* 51, no. 5 (2010): 1049–1056.

Benammi, Hind, Omar El Hiba, Abderrahmane Romane, and Halima Gamrani. "A blunted anxiolytic like effect of curcumin against acute lead induced anxiety in rat: involvement of serotonin." *Acta Histochemica* 116, no. 5 (2014): 920–925.

Bermond, P. "Therapy of side effects of oral contraceptive agents with vitamin B6." *Acta Vitaminologica et Enzymologica* 4, no. 1–2 (1981): 45–54.

Block, Gladys, Christopher D. Jensen, Tapashi B. Dalvi, Edward P. Norkus, Mark Hudes, Patricia B. Crawford, Nina Holland, Ellen B. Fung, Laurie Schumacher, and Paul Harmatz. "Vitamin C treatment reduces elevated C-reactive protein." *Free Radical Biology and Medicine* 46, no. 1 (2009): 70–77.

Brasky, Theodore M., Amy K. Darke, Xiaoling Song, Catherine M. Tangen, Phyllis J. Goodman, Ian M. Thompson, Frank L. Meyskens, et al. "Plasma phospholipid fatty acids and prostate cancer risk in the SELECT trial." *Journal of the National Cancer Institute* (2013): djt174.

Bravo, Javier A., Paul Forsythe, Marianne V. Chew, Emily Escaravage, Hélène M. Savignac, Timothy G. Dinan, John Bienenstock, and John F. Cryan. "Ingestion of Lactobacillus strain regulates emotional behavior and central GABA receptor expression in a mouse via the vagus nerve." *Proceedings of the National Academy of Sciences* 108, no. 38 (2011): 16050–16055.

Burton, J. M. "Long-term vitamin D in depression." Annual meeting of the American Academy of Neurology, April 2009.

Bystritsky, Alexander, Lauren Kerwin, and Jamie D. Feusner. "A pilot study of Rhodiola rosea (Rhodax®) for generalized anxiety disorder (GAD)." *The Journal of Alternative and Complementary Medicine* 14, no. 2 (2008): 175–180.

Chandrasekhar, K., Jyoti Kapoor, and Sridhar Anishetty. "A prospective, randomized double-blind, placebo-controlled study of safety and efficacy of a high-concentration full-spectrum extract of ashwagandha root in reducing stress and anxiety in adults." *Indian Journal of Psychological Medicine* 34, no. 3 (2012): 255.

Connor, K. M., and J. R. T. Davidson. "A placebo-controlled study of kava kava in generalized anxiety disorder." *International Clinical Psychopharmacology* 17, no. 4 (2002): 185–188.

Daniela, Jezova, Makatsori Aikaterini, Smriga Miro, Morinaga Yasushi, and Duncko Roman. "Subchronic treatment with amino acid mixture of L-lysine and L-arginine modifies neuroendocrine activation during psychosocial stress in subjects with high trait anxiety." *Nutritional Neuroscience* 8, no. 3 (2005): 155–160.

Darbinyan, V., G. Aslanyan, E. Amroyan, E. Gabrielyan, C. Malmström, and A. Panossian. "Clinical trial of Rhodiola rosea L. extract SHR-5 in the treatment of mild to moderate depression." *Nordic Journal of Psychiatry* 61, no. 5 (2007): 343–348.

Davidson, J. R., Cindy Crawford, John A. Ives, and Wayne B. Jonas. "Homeopathic treatments in psychiatry: a systematic review of randomized placebo-controlled studies." *The Journal of Clinical Psychiatry* 72, no. 6 (2011): 795–805.

Davidson, J. R., R. M. Morrison, J. Shore, R. T. Davidson, and G. Bedayn. "Homeopathic treatment of depression and anxiety." *Alternative Therapies in Health and Medicine* 3, no. 1 (1997): 46–49.

Fortmann, Stephen P., Brittany U. Burda, Caitlyn A. Senger, Jennifer S. Lin, and Evelyn P. Whitlock. "Vitamin and mineral supplements in the primary prevention of cardiovascular disease and cancer: an updated systematic evidence review for the US Preventive Services Task Force." *Annals of Internal Medicine* 159, no. 12 (2013): 824–834.

Fux, Mendel, Joseph Levine, Alex Aviv, and R. H. Belmaker. "Inositol treatment of obsessive-compulsive disorder." *The American Journal of Psychiatry* 153, no. 9 (1996): 1219–1221.

Geller, Stacie E., and Laura Studee. "Botanical and dietary supplements for mood and anxiety in menopausal women." *Menopause* 14, no. 3 (2007): 541–549.

Ghanizadeh, Ahmad, and Ebrahim Moghimi-Sarani. "A randomized double blind placebo controlled clinical trial of N-Acetylcysteine added to risperidone for treating autistic disorders." *BMC Psychiatry* 13, no. 1 (2013): 196.

Ghanizadeh, Ahmad, Nima Derakhshan, and Michael Berk. "N-acetylcysteine versus placebo for treating nail biting, a double blind randomized placebo controlled clinical trial." *Anti-Inflammatory & Anti-Allergy Agents in Medicinal Chemistry* (Formerly *Current Medicinal Chemistry-Anti-Inflammatory and Anti-Allergy Agents*) 12, no. 3 (2013): 223–228.

Gilhotra, Neeraj, and Dinesh Dhingra. "GABAergic and nitriergic modulation by curcumin for its antianxiety-like activity in mice." *Brain Research* 1352 (2010): 167–175.

Grant, Jon E., Brian L. Odlaug, and Suck Won Kim. "N-acetylcysteine, a glutamate modulator, in the treatment of trichotillomania: a double-blind, placebo-controlled study." *Archives of General Psychiatry* 66, no. 7 (2009): 756–763.

Harris, Elizabeth, Joni Kirk, Renee Rowsell, Luis Vitetta, Avni Sali, Andrew B. Scholey, and Andrew Pipingas. "The effect of multivitamin supplementation on mood and stress in healthy older men." *Human Psychopharmacology: Clinical and Experimental* 26, no. 8 (2011): 560–567.

Hellhammer, Juliane, and Melanie Schubert. "Effects of a homeopathic combination remedy on the acute stress response, well-being, and sleep: a double-blind, randomized clinical trial." *The Journal of Alternative and Complementary Medicine* 19, no. 2 (2013): 161–169.

Hoffer, A., and H. Osmond. "Malvaria: a new psychiatric disease." *Acta Psychiatrica Scandinavica* 39, no. 2 (1963): 335–366.

Husain, Gulam M., Shyam Sunder Chatterjee, P. N. Singh, and V. Kumar. "Beneficial effect of Hypericum perforatum on depression and anxiety in a type 2 diabetic rat model." *Acta Pol Pharm* 68, no. 6 (2011): 913–918.

Jacka, Felice N., Simon Overland, Robert Stewart, Grethe S. Tell, Ingvar Bjelland, and Arnstein Mykletun. "Association between magnesium intake and depression and anxiety in community-dwelling adults: the Hordaland Health Study." *Australian and New Zealand Journal of Psychiatry* 43, no. 1 (2009): 45–52.

Jorissen, B. L., F. Brouns, M. P. J. Van Boxtel, and W. J. Riedel. "Safety of soy-derived phosphatidylserine in elderly people." *Nutritional Neuroscience* 5, no. 5 (2002): 337–343.

Kahn, René S., Herman G. M. Westenberg, Wim Ma Verhoeven, Christien C. Gispen-De Wied, and Wilma D. J. Kamerbeek. "Effect of a serotonin precursor and uptake inhibitor in anxiety disorders; a double-blind comparison of 5-hydroxytryptophan, clomipramine and placebo." *International Clinical Psychopharmacology* 2, no. 1 (1987): 33–45.

Kalani, Amir, Gul Bahtiyar, and Alan Sacerdote. "Ashwagandha root in the treatment of non-classical adrenal hyperplasia." *BMJ case reports* 2012 (2012): bcr2012006989.

Katzenschlager, R., A. Evans, A. Manson, P. N. Patsalos, N. Ratnaraj, H. Watt, L. Timmermann, R. Van der Giessen, and A. J. Lees. "Mucuna pruriens in Parkinson's disease: a double blind clinical and pharmacological study." *Journal of Neurology, Neurosurgery & Psychiatry* 75, no. 12 (2004): 1672–1677.

Kiecolt-Glaser, Janice K., Martha A. Belury, Rebecca Andridge, William B. Malarkey, and Ronald Glaser. "Omega-3 supplementation lowers inflammation and anxiety in medical students: a randomized controlled trial." *Brain, Behavior, and Immunity* 25, no. 8 (2011): 1725–1734.

Lamina, S., and G. C. Okoye. "Effect of interval exercise training programme on C-reactive protein in the non-pharmacological management of hypertension: a randomized controlled trial." *African Journal of Medicine and Medical Sciences* 41, no. 4 (2012): 379–386.

Lapin, Izyaslav. "Phenibut (β-Phenyl-GABA): a tranquilizer and nootropic drug." *CNS Drug Reviews* 7, no. 4 (2001): 471–481.

Leung, Sumie, Rodney J. Croft, Barry V. O'Neill, and Pradeep J. Nathan. "Acute high-dose glycine attenuates mismatch negativity (MMN) in healthy human controls." *Psychopharmacology* 196, no. 3 (2008): 451–460.

Lewis, John E., Eduard Tiozzo, Angelica B. Melillo, Susanna Leonard, Lawrence Chen, Armando Mendez, Judi M. Woolger, and Janet Konefal. "The effect of methylated vitamin B complex on depressive and anxiety symptoms and quality of life in adults with depression." *International Scholarly Research Notices* 2013 (2013).

Liu, Joanne J., Hanga C. Galfalvy, Thomas B. Cooper, Maria A. Oquendo, Michael F. Grunebaum, J. John Mann, and M. Elizabeth Sublette. "Omega-3 polyunsaturated fatty acid status in major depression with comorbid anxiety disorders." *The Journal of Clinical Psychiatry* 74, no. 7 (2013): 732.

Long, Sara-Jayne, and David Benton. "Effects of vitamin and mineral supplementation on stress, mild psychiatric symptoms, and mood in nonclinical samples: a meta-analysis." *Psychosomatic Medicine* 75, no. 2 (2013): 144–153.

Mahdi, Abbas Ali, Kamla Kant Shukla, Mohammad Kaleem Ahmad, Singh Rajender, Satya Narain Shankhwar, Vishwajeet Singh, and Deepansh Dalela. "Withania somnifera improves semen quality in stress-related male fertility." *Evidence-Based Complementary and Alternative Medicine* 2011 (2011).

Malsch, U., and M. Kieser. "Efficacy of kava-kava in the treatment of nonpsychotic anxiety, following pretreatment with benzodiazepines." *Psychopharmacology* 157, no. 3 (2001): 277–283.

Messaoudi, Michaël, Robert Lalonde, Nicolas Violle, Hervé Javelot, Didier Desor, Amine Nejdi, Jean-François Bisson, et al. "Assessment of psychotropic-like properties of a probiotic formulation (Lactobacillus helveticus R0052 and Bifidobacterium longum R0175) in rats and human subjects." *British Journal of Nutrition* 105, no. 05 (2011): 755–764.

Misner, Bill. "Food alone may not provide sufficient micronutrients for preventing deficiency." *Journal of the International Society of Sports Nutrition* 3, no. 1 (2006): 51–6.

Miyasaka, Lincoln Sakiara, Álvaro N. Atallah, and Bernardo Soares. "Passiflora for anxiety disorder." *The Cochrane Library* (2007).

Monteleone, Palmiero, M. Maj, L. Beinat, M. Natale, and D. Kemali. "Blunting by chronic phosphatidylserine administration of the stress-induced activation of the hypothalamo-pituitary-adrenal axis in healthy men." *European Journal of Clinical Pharmacology* 42, no. 4 (1992): 385–388.

Morales, Paola, Nicola Simola, Diego Bustamante, Francisco Lisboa, Jenny Fiedler, Peter J. Gebicke-Haerter, Micaela Morelli, R. Andrew Tasker, and Mario Herrera-Marschitz. "Nicotinamide prevents the long-term effects of perinatal asphyxia on apoptosis, non-spatial working memory and anxiety in rats." *Experimental Brain Research* 202, no. 1 (2010): 1–14.

Morris, N. "The effects of lavender (Lavendula angustifolium) baths on psychological well-being: two exploratory randomised control trials." *Complementary Therapies in Medicine* 10, no. 4 (2002): 223–228.

Movafegh, Ali, Reza Alizadeh, Fatimah Hajimohamadi, Fatimah Esfehani, and Mohmad Nejatfar. "Preoperative oral Passiflora incarnata reduces anxiety in ambulatory surgery patients: a double-blind, placebo-controlled study." *Anesthesia & Analgesia* 106, no. 6 (2008): 1728–1732.

O'Neill, Barry V., Rodney J. Croft, Sumie Leung, Chris Oliver, K. Luan Phan, and Pradeep J. Nathan. "High-dose glycine inhibits the loudness dependence of the auditory evoked potential (LDAEP) in healthy humans." *Psychopharmacology* 195, no. 1 (2007): 85–93.

Pilkington, Karen, Graham Kirkwood, Hagen Rampes, Peter Fisher, and Janet Richardson. "Homeopathy for depression: a systematic review of the research evidence." *Homeopathy* 94, no. 3 (2005): 153–163.

Poyares, Dalva R., Christian Guilleminault, Maurice M. Ohayon, and Sergio Tufik. "Can valerian improve the sleep of insomniacs after benzodiazepine withdrawal?" *Progress in Neuro-Psychopharmacology and Biological Psychiatry* 26, no. 3 (2002): 539–545.

Presser, A. "Herb-drug interactions presentation at the University of Southern California School of Pharmacy." Natural Products Association, Las Vegas, 2005.

Quinlan, John F. "Hypoglycemia: in relation to the anxiety states and the degenerative diseases." *California and Western Medicine* 49, no. 6 (1938): 446.

Rao, A. Venket, Alison C. Bested, Tracey M. Beaulne, Martin A. Katzman, Christina Iorio, John M. Berardi, and Alan C. Logan. "A randomized, double-blind, placebo-controlled pilot study of a probiotic in emotional symptoms of chronic fatigue syndrome." *Gut Pathogens* 1, no. 1 (2009): 1–6.

Ridaura, Vanessa K., Jeremiah J. Faith, Federico E. Rey, Jiye Cheng, Alexis E. Duncan, Andrew L. Kau, Nicholas W. Griffin, et al. "Gut microbiota from twins discordant for obesity modulate metabolism in mice." *Science* 341, no. 6150 (2013): 1241214.

Russo, A. J. "Decreased zinc and increased copper in individuals with anxiety." *Nutrition and Metabolic Insights* 4 (2011): 1.

Sánchez-Villegas, A., J. Doreste, J. Schlatter, J. Pla, M. Bes-Rastrollo, and M. A. Martínez-González. "Association between folate, vitamin B6 and vitamin B12 intake and depression in the SUN cohort study." *Journal of Human Nutrition and Dietetics* 22, no. 2 (2009): 122–133.

Schruers, Koen, Rob van Diest, Thea Overbeek, and Eric Griez. "Acute L-5-hydroxytryptophan administration inhibits carbon dioxide-induced panic in panic disorder patients." *Psychiatry Research* 113, no. 3 (2002): 237–243.

Shao, L., J. Cui, L. T. Young, and J. F. Wang. "The effect of mood stabilizer lithium on expression and activity of glutathione s-transferase isoenzymes." *Neuroscience* 151, no. 2 (2008): 518–524.

Shrivastava, Sandeep, Thomas J. Pucadyil, Yamuna Devi Paila, Sourav Ganguly, and Amitabha Chattopadhyay. "Chronic cholesterol depletion using statin impairs the function and dynamics of human serotonin1A receptors." *Biochemistry* 49, no. 26 (2010): 5426–5435.

Sommerfield, Andrew J., Ian J. Deary, and Brian M. Frier. "Acute hyperglycemia alters mood state and impairs cognitive performance in people with type 2 diabetes." *Diabetes Care* 27, no. 10 (2004): 2335–2340.

Stough, Con, Andrew Scholey, Jenny Lloyd, Jo Spong, Stephen Myers, and Luke A. Downey. "The effect of 90 day administration of a high dose vitamin B-complex on work stress." *Human Psychopharmacology: Clinical and Experimental* 26, no. 7 (2011): 470–476.

Teschke, Rolf, Alexander Schwarzenboeck, and Ahmet Akinci. "Kava hepatotoxicity: a European view." *The New Zealand Medical Journal* 121, no. 1283 (2008): 90–98.

Thorne Research, Inc. "Phosphatidylserine." *Alternative Medicine Review* 13, no. 3 (2008).

U.S. Food and Drug Administration. "Consumer advisory: kava-containing dietary supplements may be associated with severe liver injury." (2013).

Winstock, A. R., T. Lea, and J. Copeland. "Lithium carbonate in the management of cannabis withdrawal in humans: an open-label study." *Journal of Psychopharmacology* (2008).

Witte, Steffen, Dieter Loew, and Wilhelm Gaus. "Meta-analysis of the efficacy of the acetonic kava-kava extract WS® 1490 in patients with nonpsychotic anxiety disorders." *Phytotherapy Research* 19, no. 3 (2005): 183–188.

Woelk, H., and S. Schläfke. "A multi-center, double-blind, randomised study of the Lavender oil preparation Silexan in comparison to Lorazepam for generalized anxiety disorder." *Phytomedicine* 17, no. 2 (2010): 94–99.

Yoto, A., S. Murao, M. Motoki, Y. Yokoyama, N. Horie, K. Takeshima, K. Masuda, M. Kim, and H. Yokogoshi. "Oral intake of γ-aminobutyric acid affects mood and activities of central nervous system during stressed condition induced by mental tasks." *Amino Acids* 43, no. 3 (2012): 1331–1337.

Yoto, Ai, Mao Motoki, Sato Murao, and Hidehiko Yokogoshi. "Effects of L-theanine or caffeine intake on changes in blood pressure under physical and psychological stresses." *Journal of Physiological Anthropology* 31 (2012): 28.

Zheng, Ju-Sheng, Xiao-Jie Hu, Yi-Min Zhao, Jing Yang, and Duo Li. "Intake of fish and marine n-3 polyunsaturated fatty acids and risk of breast cancer: meta-analysis of data from 21 independent prospective cohort studies." *BMJ* 346 (2013).

index

massage to lower, 104
naturopathic medicine to lower, 92, 94
serotonin syndrome and, 130
stress and, 11
taurine to lower, 127
theanine to lower, 127, 128
vitamin C to lower, 189
yoga to lower, 100, 101
blood sugar
balancing, 4–5
diary, 82
digestive health and, 81–83
sleep deprivation and, 27–28
steps to improve, 82
blood tests, 2, 169–184
ABO blood type, 172
blood sugar panel, 171
blood work list, 170
CBC, 171
celiac panel, 180–181
cholesterol panel, 172
CMP, 171
hormonal panel, 175–180
inflammation panel, 172–174
iron panel, 174
for lithium levels, 122
nutrient panel, 181–184
blood type diet, 78, 79, 172, 195
Bongiorno, Peter, 139, 196
books for new messages, 15–16
botanical medicines. *See* herbal supplements
brain, stress system and, 9–11
brain cell destruction, 97
brain cell regeneration
exercise for, 45
meditation for, 97
brain-derived neurotrophic factor (BDNF), 44, 58, 111, 120–121, 122
breakfast ideas
Dr. Peter's gluten-free waffles, 200
Greek yogurt sundae, 200
Inner Source Cleanse smoothie, 199–200
nut butter on sprouted toast, 199
poached eggs on sprouted bread, 199
quick oatmeal, 199
breathing
deep, in mind-body therapy, 96–99
for healthy digestive tract, 54

Buddhism, 20–23
Buddhism for Beginners (Chodron), 22–23
Buspar (Buspirone), 159
B vitamins, 115–118
B complex, 116–117
folic acid (folate), 116, 117
food sources of, 117–118
inositol, 116, 117
toxicity, 117
vitamin B3 (niacinamide), 115
vitamin B6 (pyridoxine), 115
vitamin B12 (methylcobalamin), 115–116

cadmium, 190–191
calcarea carbonica, 154
Campbell, Joseph, 7, 12–13, 15, 16
Carex Daylight Classic (DL930), 196
catechol-o-methyltransferase (COMT), 184–185
CBC. *See* complete blood count (CBC)
CBT. *See* cognitive behavioral therapy (CBT)
Celexa (Citalopram), 159
celiac disease, 52, 77, 180–181
Centers for Disease Control
on obesity, 60
on sleep disorders, 27
on toxins, 190
cerebral cortex, 9, 10, 86, 186
checklist for restorative sleep, 40
checkup, 1–2
chelation process, 192
chewing, for healthy digestive tract, 54–55
Chinese medicine, 39
Chinese qi gong, 97
Chlordiazepoxide (Librium), 160
Chödrön, Pema, 15, 161, 163
Chodron, Thubten, 22–23
cholesterol, 11, 43, 65, 172, 173
chromium, 119
circadian rhythm, 88–89
Citalopram (Celexa), 159
Clonazepam (Klonopin), 107, 160
Clorazepate (Tranxene), 160
CMP. *See* complete metabolic panel (CMP)
coffea cruda, 154
coffee, 69–72

about the author

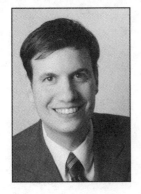

Books by Peter Bongiorno

How Come They're Happy and I'm Not? The Complete Natural Program to Healing Depression for Good. San Francisco, CA: Conari Press, 2012.

Healing Depression: Integrated Naturopathic and Conventional Treatments. Toronto, Canada: CCNM Press, 2010.

Holistic Solutions for Anxiety & Depression in Therapy: Combining Natural Remedies with Conventional Care. New York: W.W. Norton, 2015.

Contact Information for Dr. Peter Bongiorno

www.drpeterbongiorno.com
www.InnerSourceHealth.com
info@innersourcehealth.com

Twitter:
  @drbongiorno
  @InnerSourceH

Facebook:
  www.facebook.com/peter.bongiorno
  www.facebook.com/pages/InnerSource-Health/200391990434

***Psychology Today* blog:**
  www.psychologytoday.com/experts/peter-bongiorno-nd-lac

Mailing Address:
  Inner Source Health
  345 7th Avenue, 16th floor
  New York, NY 10001

Join Dr. Peter Bongiorno's clinic newsletter at the bottom of the homepage at *www.InnerSourceHealth.com*.

to our readers

Conari Press, an imprint of Red Wheel/Weiser, publishes books on topics ranging from spirituality, personal growth, and relationships to women's issues, parenting, and social issues. Our mission is to publish quality books that will make a difference in people's lives—how we feel about ourselves and how we relate to one another. We value integrity, compassion, and receptivity, both in the books we publish and in the way we do business.

Our readers are our most important resource, and we appreciate your input, suggestions, and ideas about what you would like to see published.

Visit our website at *www.redwheelweiser.com* to learn about our upcoming books and free downloads, and be sure to go to *www.redwheelweiser.com/newsletter* to sign up for newsletters and exclusive offers.

You can also contact us at *info@rwwbooks.com*.

Conari Press
an imprint of Red Wheel/Weiser, LLC
665 Third Street, Suite 400
San Francisco, CA 94107